GET FIT NOW FOR

HIGH SCHOOL
FOOTBALL

STEWART SMITH AND
CHRIS JOHNSON

PHOTOGRAPHY BY
PETER FIELD PECK

A GETFITNOW.COM BOOK
Hatherleigh Press, New York

GetFitNow.com Books
An Independent Imprint of Hatherleigh Press

Hatherleigh Press/GetFitNow.com Books
5-22 46th Avenue Ste 200
Long Island City, NY 11101
1-800-367-2550
www.getfitnow.com

Before beginning any strenuous exercise program consult your physician. The author and publisher of this book and workout disclaim any liability, personal or professional, resulting from the misapplication of any of the training procedures described in this publication.

All GetFitNow.com books are available for bulk purchase, special promotions, and premiums. For more information, please contact the manager of our Special Sales department at 1-800-367-2550.

Library of Congress Information available upon request

Photographed by Peter Field Peck
with Canon cameras and lenses on Fuji color negative film

10 9 8 7 6 5 4 3 2 1
Printed in Canada on acid-free paper.

TABLE OF CONTENTS

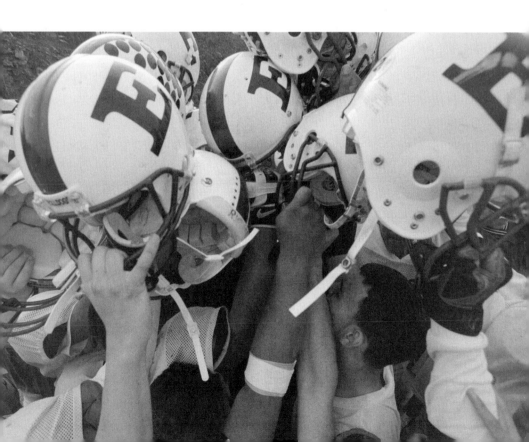

ACKNOWLEDGEMENTS

Thank you to the Union City Board of Education and the Emerson High School Athletic Department for allowing us to photograph the Emerson High School football team in action for this book.

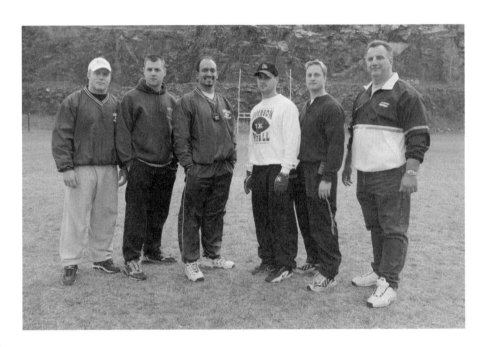

Thank you also to the players and coaches for their enthusiasm during the photo shoot, and for allowing us to observe their hard work in practice and the weight room.

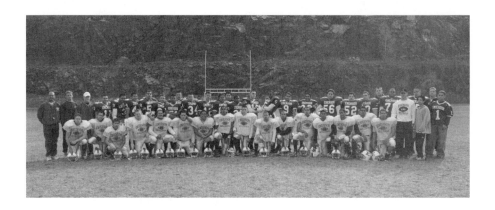

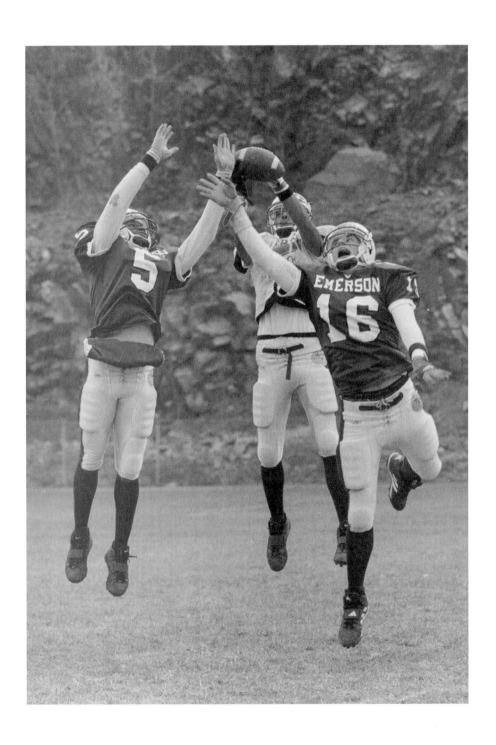

DEDICATION

This book is dedicated to the hundreds of thousands of high school football players across the nation who dedicate their time and energy to getting bigger, faster and stronger. We hope this book contributes to your next winning season!

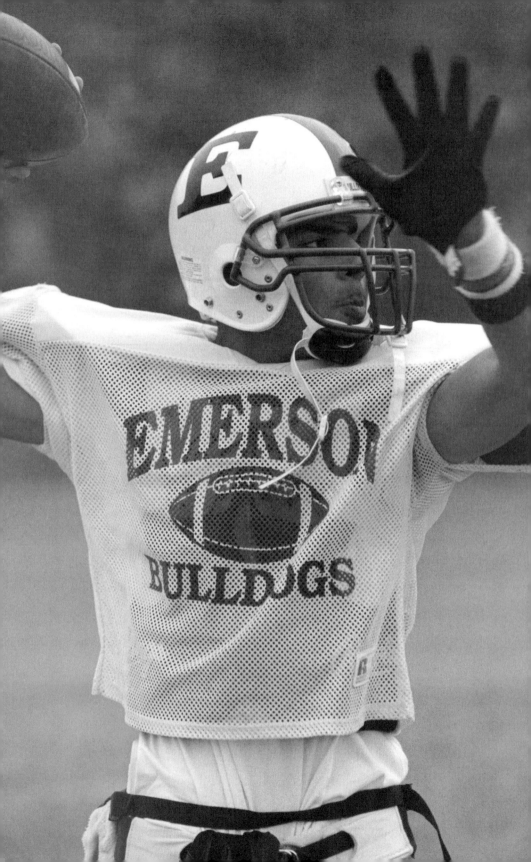

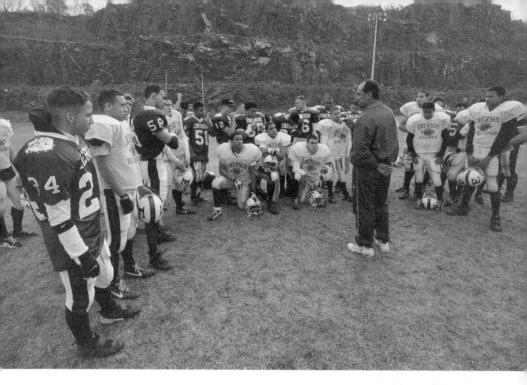

CHAPTER 1:

INTRODUCTION

Every year thousands of high school students across the country decide to play football. Some of these students have experience with organized football; others have no experience at all.

If you already have a year or two of high school football under your belt, you know that football at the high school level is very different from anything you've tried before. The speed of the game is faster, the contact is more aggressive, the players are bigger, and the mental game plays a critical role. To compete at this level, you'll need to be in the best shape of your life and have a true commitment to winning. You'll need to workout consistently both during the season and during the off-season, memorize plays, practice drills, and lift weights. For the first time, competition plays a key role. The only way to ensure that you're at your best is if you work harder than the competition. For most players, high school sports represent the first time your sole goal in competing is WINNING.

So, why would anyone want to endure long practices, sore muscles, and mental stress to play high school football? If you have to think too hard about the answer to that, you should re-evaluate your commitment!

High school football will help shape the person you become. How?

TEAMWORK

In order to ensure victory, eleven people must work in unison to accomplish the goal—every play. You're dependent on the person next to you, the person behind you, and the people on the sideline.

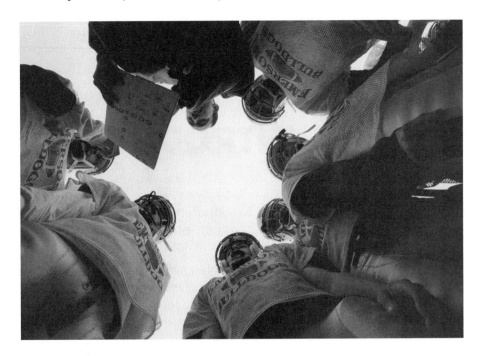

DISCIPLINE

There are many rules to be followed in football to ensure success! This includes the rules of the game, the rules of the coaches, how you treat your fellow players and the opponents, and your own personal discipline in working out and committing to the team. A high level of discipline is required, because people are counting on you.

CAMARADERIE

Because you spend so much time with the people on your team, you will develop friendships that can be lifelong. Everyone on the team shares victory parties!

LEADERSHIP

There's going to come a time when someone has to step up and lead others. It might be the most important play of the game, or just a practice that doesn't seem to be going well. Being a leader on the field will help you be a leader off the field.

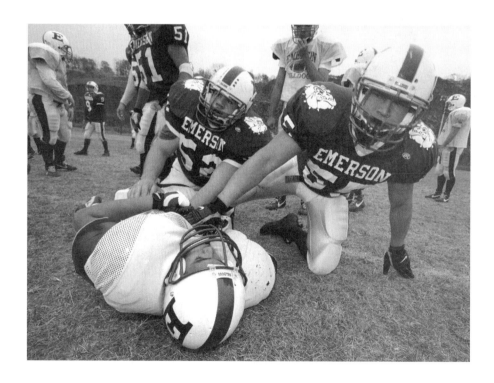

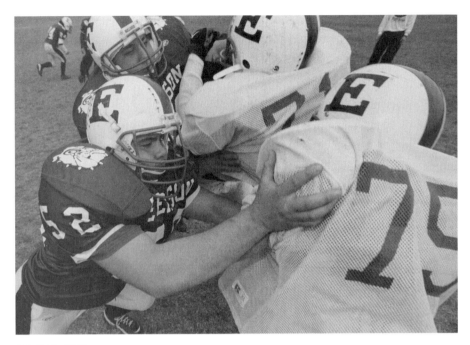

HUMILITY

It's a fact: you will win big games, and you will lose big games. How you choose to act in victory and defeat is a true reflection of your character.

In addition, you will have your own personal reasons for playing, from the chance of a scholarship to college, to the sheer fun of it.

PREPARING FOR FOOTBALL SEASON

If the first time you workout is the first day of practice, you will be in big trouble both physically and mentally. Every good football player knows that one of the keys to success is a consistent commitment to an off-season workout. Though the season only technically lasts for four months, the commitment is year-round.

This book is designed to walk you through the steps to make you a quality football player. We haven't focused in this book on working out during the season—your coaches will certainly keep you busy in that respect. We have focused on the basic calisthenics, weight lifting exercises, agility drills and conditioning that you will need to prepare for success during the season. Remember, it is critical to have a good balance between conditioning, weight lifting and drills. While it might be tempting to stay in the weight room all summer and work on getting bigger, this won't help you on the field unless you are faster and able to sustain your strength throughout the game as well.

A key to success is staying flexible and adapting your routine to your personal objectives. The exercises in this book and the workout are not geared toward any specific positions, partially because many high school football players try multiple positions as their bodies and abilities change during the four years. Equally, many high school players play at multiple positions (offensive and defensive lines, for example). At the next level of football, your focus will be on one specific position, and the workouts are more targeted to the needs of that position. However, even at the high school level, you may want to tailor your workout to your own needs and fitness level, and you should feel comfortable doing so. Always consult with your coach or your doctor when starting any new workout, or significantly increasing your exercise levels.

Football is one of the most strenuous physical sports, requiring the ability to hit hard, think fast, and have endurance for the whole game. Winning on the football field is one of the best feelings in the world—and losing one of the worst. To make sure you are ready to win this season, start now. Good luck!

A NOTE ABOUT NUTRITION

All the working out in the world won't help you at all unless you concentrate on eating healthy as well. Good nutrition promotes vital muscle and tissue growth and repair. The ideal diet provides all the nutrients that the body needs and supplies energy for exercise. A high carbohydrate diet is essential to maintaining energy during successive days of heavy training, but this should not include foods high in fat. Remember, while carbohydrates and proteins produce only 4 calories per gram, fat provides the body with 9 calories per gram.

You should also remember that frequent water intake is crucial. Drink at least four quarts of water daily, and stay away from alcohol or tobacco, which increase your body's need for water. (Smoking is a sure sign that you are not committed to football, and will definitely affect your ability to give 110% the whole game.)

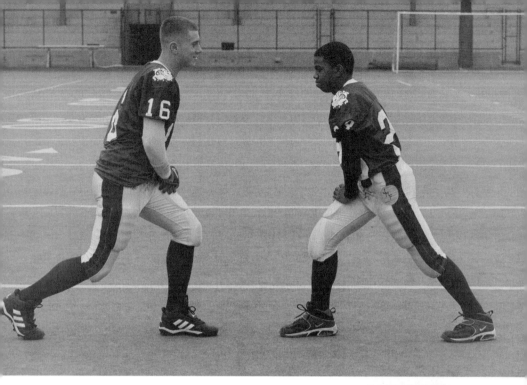

CHAPTER 2:

STRETCHING

Stretching may not seem very important. It certainly isn't the most tiring part of the workout and it's not difficult. It may seem that stretching is just killing time before the real workout begins. Yet don't be fooled. Stretching exercises should start and end every workout, for a number of reasons:

• Stretching before you work out helps prevent injury by warming up your muscles, tendons, and ligaments, minimizing the risk of overextension.

• Stretching before your workout actually lets you train harder. By warming up your body, you are making sure that your muscles aren't stiff or inflexible, giving you the ability to get more from your workout.

• Stretching helps increase overall flexibility—a great advantage for almost every position in football.

Stretch for about ten minutes before your workout, and about ten to fifteen minutes after your workout. Stretches should be performed slowly, and positions should be held for approximately 15 seconds (for 2 reps) unless otherwise noted.

PRE/POST WORKOUT STRETCHING ROUTINE

You may want to start your stretching routine with a quick lap around the track (about a 1/4 mile).

STRETCH	TIME
Neck rotations (2 variations)	30 seconds each variation
Arm and shoulder stretches (2 variations)	30 seconds each arm, each variation
Alternating arm circles	30 seconds each arm
Chest stretch	30 seconds
Abdominal stretches (2 variations)	30 seconds each variation
Lower back stretch	30 seconds
Groin stretch	30 seconds
ITB stretches (2 variations)	30 seconds each leg, each variation
Thigh stretch	30 seconds each leg
Toe touches	30 seconds
Calf stretches (2 variations)	30 seconds each, each variation
Hamstring	30 seconds
Jumping jacks	1 to 2 minutes

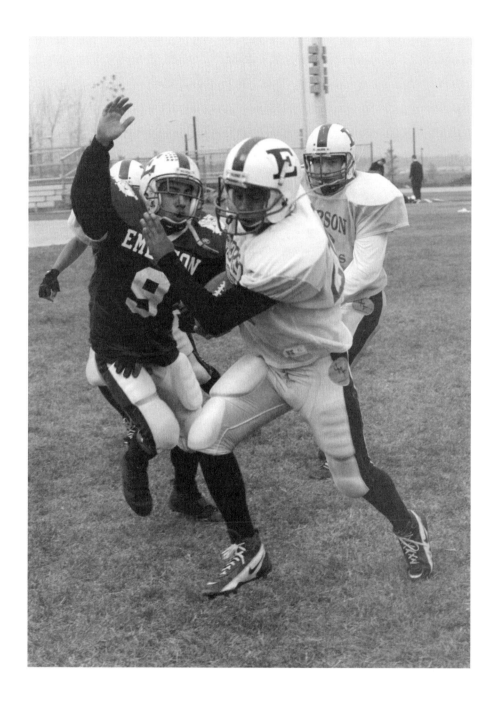

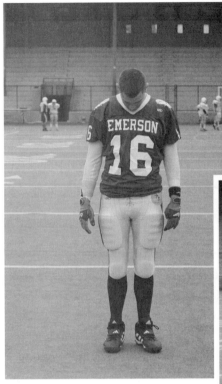

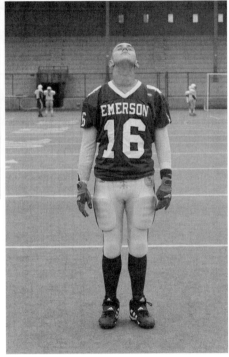

NECK ROTATIONS—FRONT TO BACK

Relax your neck muscles and move your head slowly up and down as shown. On the down movement, try to touch your chin to your chest.

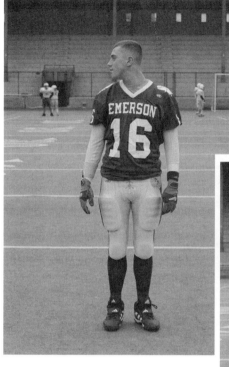

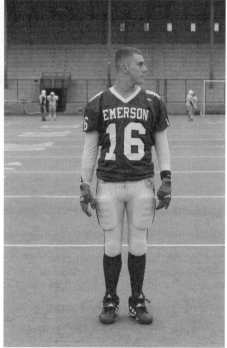

NECK ROTATIONS —SIDE TO SIDE

Relax your neck muscles and move your head slowly to the left and right as shown. Try to touch your ear to your shoulder on each movement, but try not to move your shoulders.

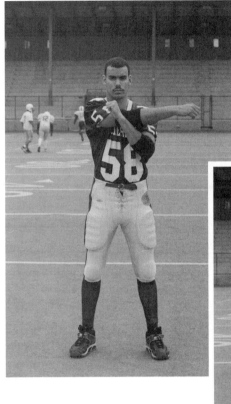

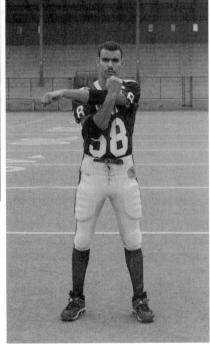

ARM AND SHOULDER STRETCH #1

With your left hand, grab your right arm at the elbow and pull it across your body. Try not to swivel your torso while doing this stretch, but concentrate on stretching your arm and shoulder. Reverse.

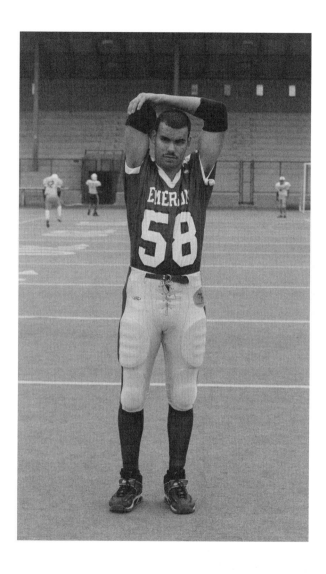

ARM AND SHOULDER STRETCH #2

Extend your arms over your head. With your left hand, grab your right arm at the elbow. Pull your elbow down until you feel the stretch in your arm, shoulder and back. You can also add to this stretch by leaning to the opposite side as you pull, stretching your abs as well. Reverse.

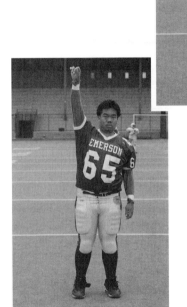

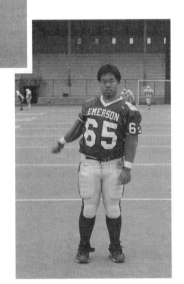

ALTERNATING ARM CIRCLES

One arm at a time, move your arm in a windmill-like movement, starting with your arm at your side and moving it forward over your head and back down again as shown.

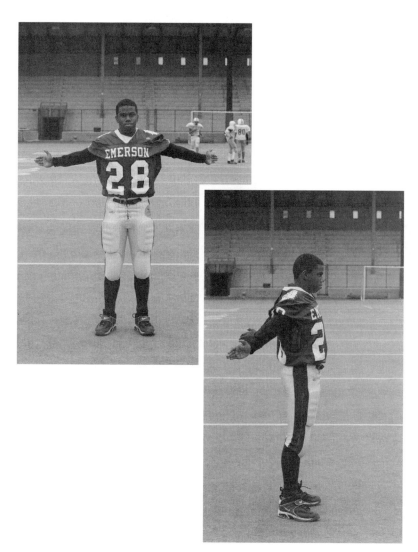

CHEST STRETCH

Extend your arms out straight to the sides at about shoulder height. Slowly press your arms backward, feeling the muscles in your chest stretch. Keep your back straight and your chest bowed.

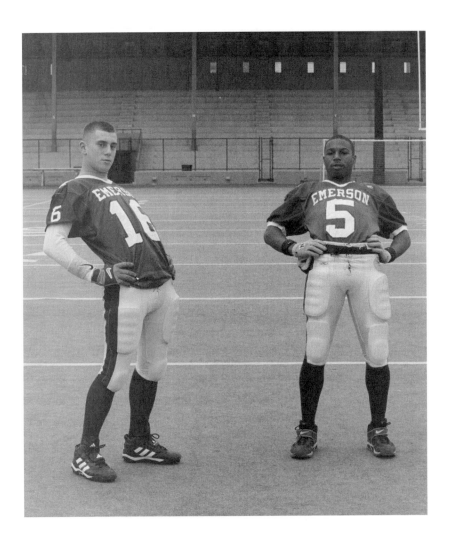

STANDING ABDOMINAL STRETCH

With your hands on your waist, slowly lean backward by pushing your hips forward and slightly arching your back. You should feel your abdominal muscles stretch as you are doing this.

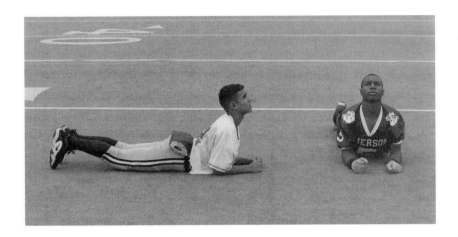

PRONE ABDOMINAL STRETCH (SNAKE)

There should be no doubt why this one is called a snake. Lie on your stomach and place your elbows under your chest as shown. Slowly lift your head and shoulders up, stretching your abdominal muscles.

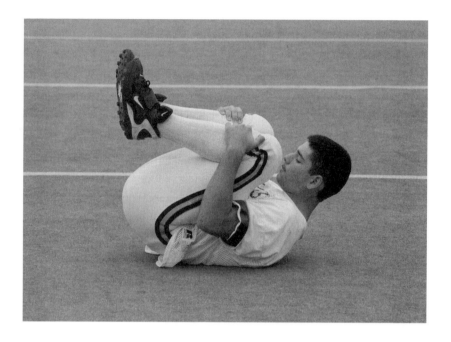

CHEST TO KNEES

Lay on your back. Bring your knees to your chest and your head toward your knees. You should feel the stretch in your lower back. You may want to try gently rocking to feel additional stretching, but be careful not to rock too aggressively.

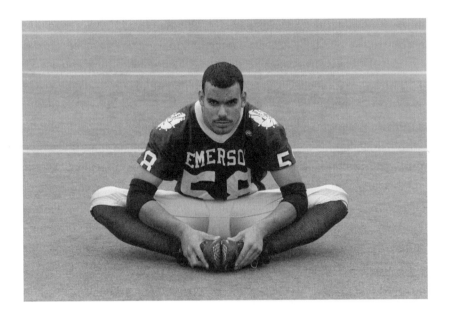

BUTTERFLY

Sit on the floor with both legs bent outward and the soles of your feet touching each other as shown. Grab your ankles with your hands and push down on your thighs with your elbows.

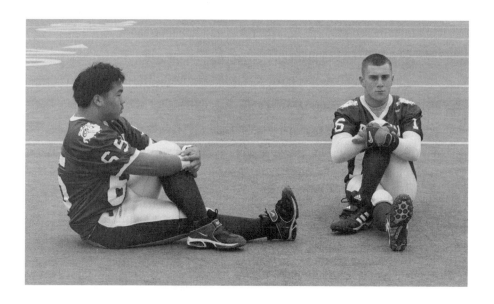

ITB STRETCH (ILIO TIBIAL BAND)

Sit on the floor with both legs extended in front of you. Cross your right leg over your left. Bend and pull your right leg to your chest as shown and hold for 15 seconds. Switch and repeat.

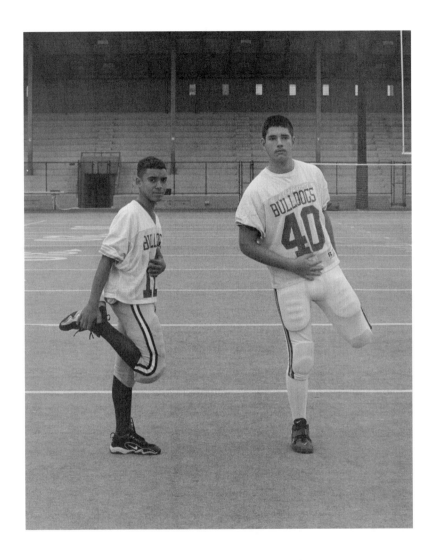

STANDING THIGH STRETCH

Stand on your left leg. Grab your right foot behind you and pull it to your buttocks. Try to keep both knees together. Hold for 15 seconds, and then switch and repeat. Do 2 reps of this stretch.

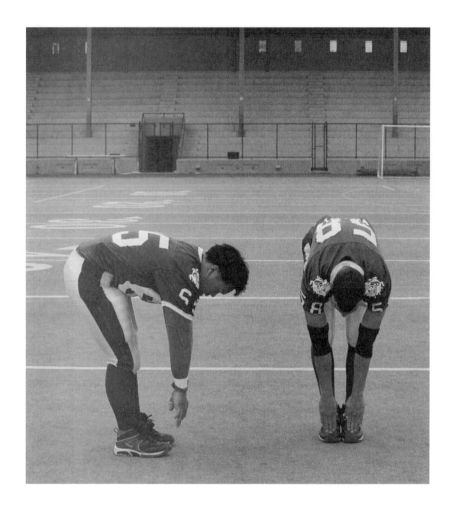

STANDING HAMSTRING STRETCH

With your feet together, bend at the waist and touch your toes. Try to keep your knees straight. Hold for 15 seconds, then repeat. This stretch can also be done with your legs spread apart, stretching your hamstrings and lower back. You can also do this stretch sitting on the floor.

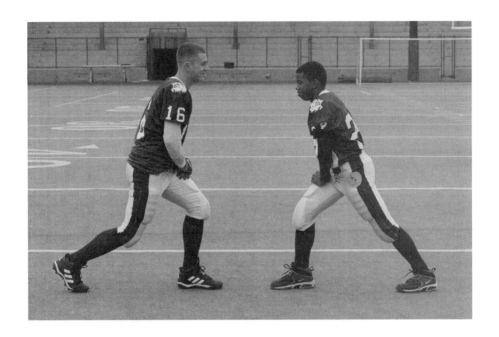

GASTROCNEMIUS (CALF) STRETCH (RIGHT PLAYER)

Stand about four feet away from sturdy, stationary object such as a wall. With most of your weight on one leg, keep that leg straight and lean into the sturdy object. Hold for about 15 seconds – switch legs and repeat. You should feel a stretch in your calf muscle from just below the back of your knee down to your Achilles tendon.

SOLEUS (ACHILLES TENDON) STRETCH (LEFT PLAYER)

Same stance as the Gastrocnemius Stretch, but bend your back knee slightly. You will feel the stretch below your calf in the Achilles tendon. Hold for 15 seconds – switch legs and repeat.

It should be noted that an Achilles tendon tear is agonizing and requires a lengthy recovery period. NFL quarterback Vinny Testaverde of the NY Jets and Hall of Fame linebacker Lawrence Taylor of the NY Giants both sustained Achilles tendon tears.

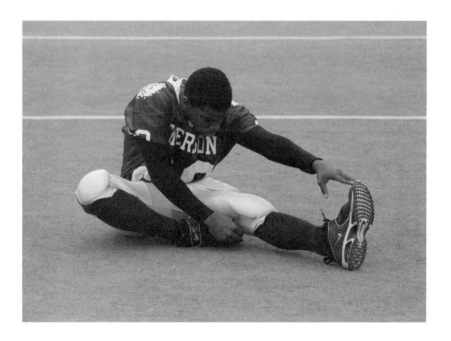

HURDLER STRIDE

Sit on the floor with legs extended in front of you. Bend right knee and place the sole of your right foot against the inside of your left knee. Lean forward toward your extended leg and grasp lower leg, ankle or foot depending on your flexibility. Hold stretch for 15 seconds. Switch legs and repeat.

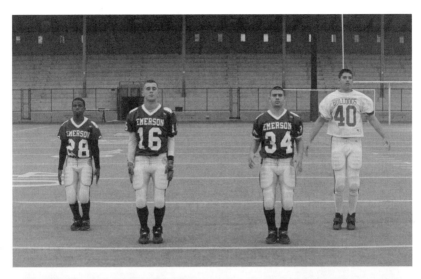

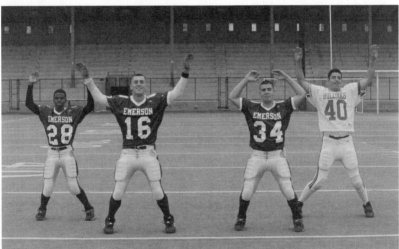

JUMPING JACKS

Standing with hands by your sides and feet together, jump up and spread your legs while simultaneously placing your arms over your head. Repeat for one minute.

It should be noted that jumping jacks can be performed in sets and reps, and may be counted in various ways (1-2-3, 1, 1-2-3, 2 etc...).

TANDEM STRETCHES

If you train with a partner (which is suggested for safety reasons) you may want to try some of these tandem stretches. You will generally find that with the assistance of your partner you will usually get a more thorough stretch.

Additionally, many high school football coaches and trainers will employ lots of tandem stretches because football equipment can be quite cumbersome and interfere with a stretch.

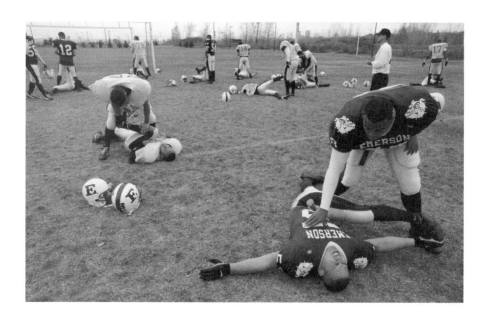

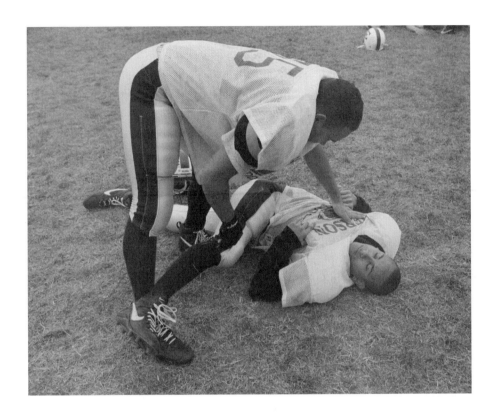

TANDEM LOWER BACK STRETCH

Partner 1 lies on back. Keeping your shoulders and hips pinned to ground rotate one leg over the other as shown. Partner 2 assists in the stretch by applying light pressure and weight to partner 1's shoulder and knee. Switch legs and repeat. You should feel a stretch in your lower back just above your buttocks.

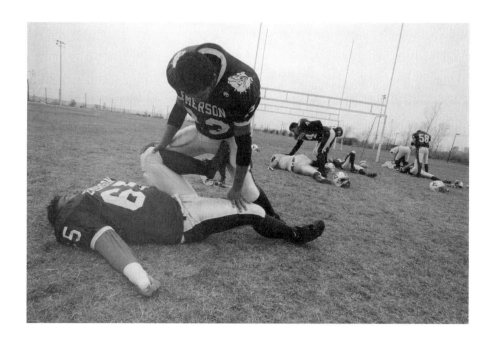

TANDEM LOWER BACK AND HIP STRETCH

Partner 1 lies on back. Lift right knee towards chest. Partner 2 grasps partner's ankle while applying light pressure and weight to partner 1's knee in a downward motion. Partner 1 should feel a lower back and hip stretch. Switch legs and repeat.

You may vary this stretch by bringing both knees into your chest while your partner applies light pressure and weight downward on both knees.

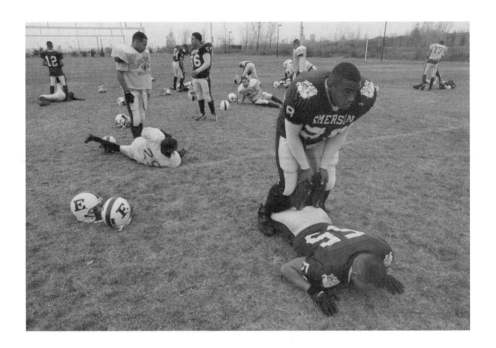

TANDEM DOUBLE QUADRICEPS STRETCH

Partner 1 lies on his stomach. Partner 2 grasps partner 1's ankles and lifts them towards buttocks while applying light weight. Partner 1 should feel thorough stretch through quadriceps area. You may also choose to stretch one leg at a time.

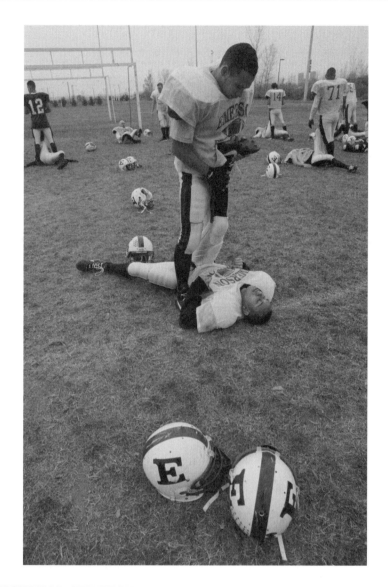

HAMSTRING STRETCH

Partner 1 lies on his back and lifts right leg. Partner 2 grasps partner 1's ankle and lifts/pushes partner 1's leg towards his head. Partner 1 must not bend his knee at all. When partner 1 begins to feel a thorough stretch partner 2 should simply hold the leg in place. Depending on your flexibility, partner may be able to push your leg past your head.

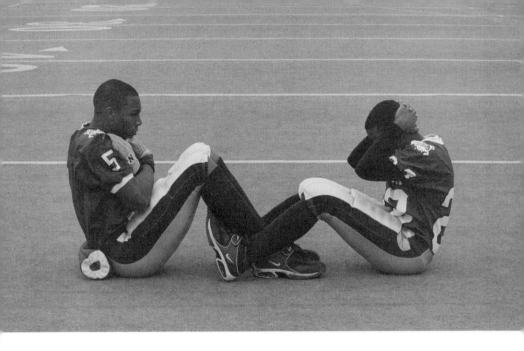

CHAPTER 3:
CALISTHENICS

Calisthenics promote good physical fitness, and help to tone and strengthen your body. Performing calisthenics is also a great way to exercise your entire body on those days when you are not weight training. By elevating your body temperature and heart rate, calisthenics can also be a great warm-up before lifting or running. Always make sure to stretch first.

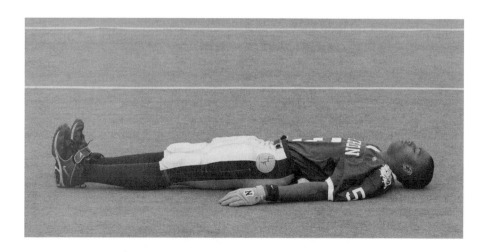

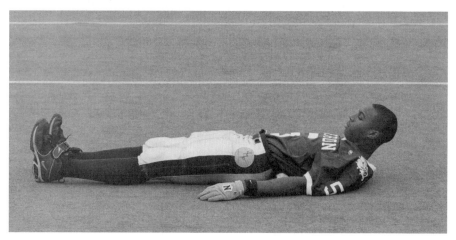

NECK EXERCISES

Lay on your back. Lift your head off the floor and move it up and down for the specified number of repetitions. You can also vary this exercise by moving your neck side to side, strengthening different neck muscles. While this may seem a simple exercise, neck injuries are very common in football, so don't skip this one.

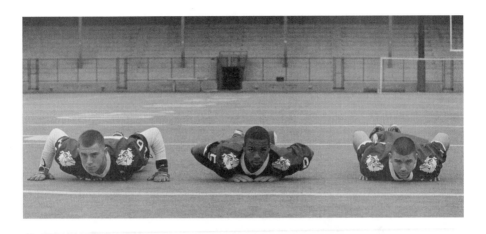

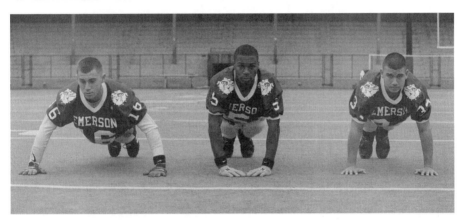

PUSH-UPS (WIDE, CLOSE AND REGULAR)

Varying the spacing of your hands when performing push-ups helps to work different muscles in your chest. Wide push-ups work your outer chest muscles, while close pushups work the triceps and inner chest more.

All push-ups are performed the same. Place the palms of your hands on the ground, keeping your feet together and your back straight. Push your body up until your arms are straight. Touch chest to the ground each repetition.

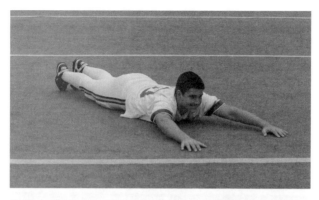

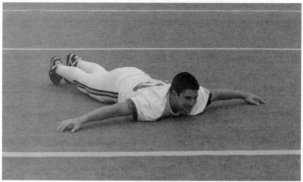

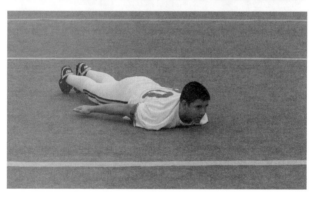

ARM HAULERS

Lay on your stomach with your back arched slightly and your head looking forward. Move your arms from the starting position over your head to your side (the movement should look almost like you are swimming). Keep your feet off the ground as well if you can. This exercise works the shoulders, lower back and buttocks, and is a favorite in the military.

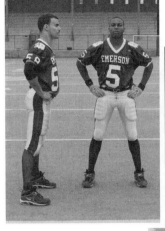

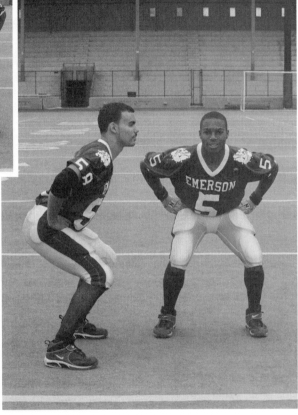

SQUATS

Place your feet about shoulder width apart. Keep your back straight and your eyes looking up. Lower yourself to a squatting position by bending your legs almost 90 degrees at the knees. Slowly raise yourself after you have reached about a sitting position. This exercise is great for the buttocks, hamstrings and quadriceps. The calisthenics version is a good alternative for using weights on the days when you aren't lifting, or as a warm-up before you lift.

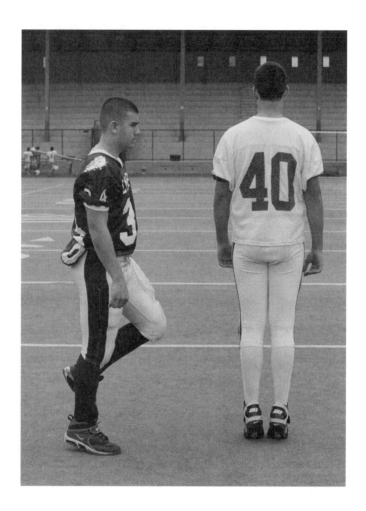

CALF AND HEEL RAISES

You can perform this exercise standing on one leg or with your feet together. If you stand on one leg, however, each muscle you are working will be isolated more. Lift yourself up onto the balls of your feet by flexing the ankle joint and calf muscle. This exercise works your calf muscles. Wide receivers, running backs, defensive backs and linebackers will benefit in particular from strong calf muscles, due to the type and amount of running they do during the game.

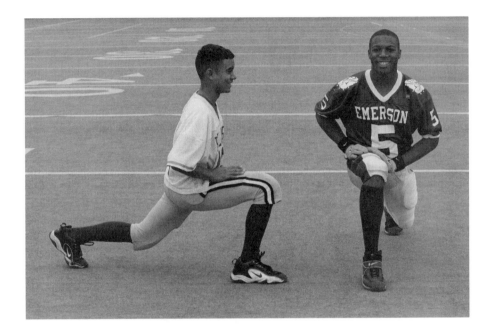

LUNGES

Take a big step forward with either leg. Lower your body by bending your knees and almost touching one knee to the floor. Switch legs and repeat. Lunges help to warm up and work out your quadriceps, hips and buttocks.

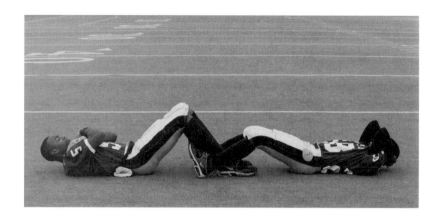

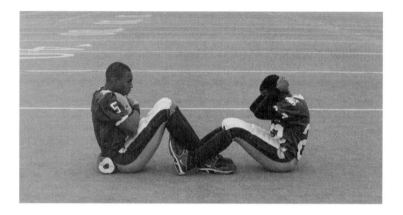

PARTNER SIT-UPS

Lay on your backs feet to feet, knees slightly bent. Interlock your feet inside partner's calf area. This will provide the support needed to lift your torso. Cross your arms over your chest or interlock your hands behind your head (both ways are shown above). Raise your upper body off the floor by contracting your stomach muscles. Raise your torso to approximately a 45 degree angle (or until your elbows touch your thighs) and repeat. Make sure you touch your shoulder blades to the floor after each repetition.

Partner sit-ups can be performed at the same time or in alternating fashion.

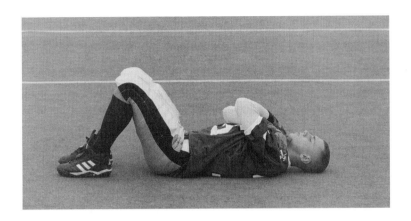

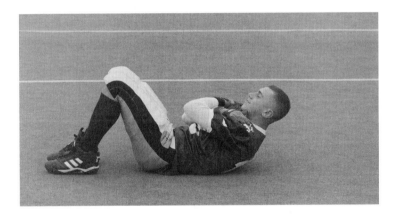

SIT-UPS

Lay on your back, knees slightly bent. Cross your arms over your chest or interlock your hands behind your head. Raise your upper body off the floor by contracting your stomach muscles. Raise your torso to approximately a 45 degree angle (or until your elbows touch your thighs) and repeat. Make sure you touch your shoulder blades to the floor after each repetition

You may also choose to do a Half Sit-up or Crunch by lifting your torso so your lower back just slightly comes off the floor.

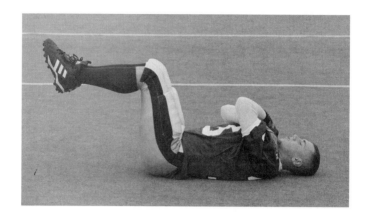

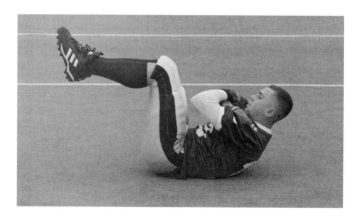

CRUNCHES

Lay on your back with your legs up in the air and bent at the knees, forming a 90-degree angle with your legs. Cross your arms over your chest. Bring your elbows to your knees slowly. DO NOT PUT YOUR HANDS BEHIND YOUR NECK AND PULL ON YOUR NECK.

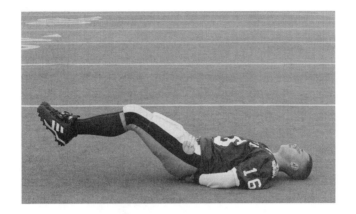

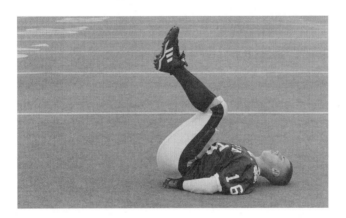

REVERSE CRUNCHES

Lay on your back with your legs up in the air and bent at the knees, forming a 90-degree angle with your legs. Bring your knees to your elbows, lifting your lower back and buttocks off the ground. Keep your upper body still and do not rock.

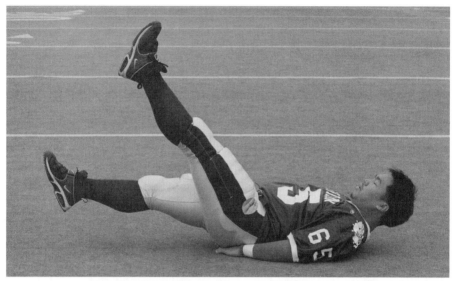

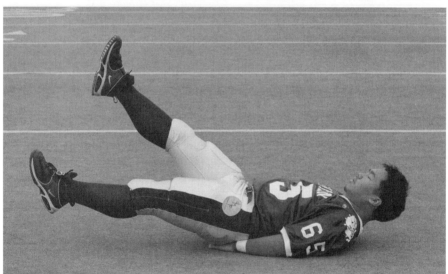

FLUTTER KICKS

Lay on your back and place your hands under your hips. Lift legs six inches off the ground and begin "walking," raising each leg approximately 3 feet off the ground. Keep your legs straight and constantly moving. With each step that you take, count 1, so the sequence will go as follows: 1,2,3 – 1; 1,2,3 – 2...for the specified number of repetitions.

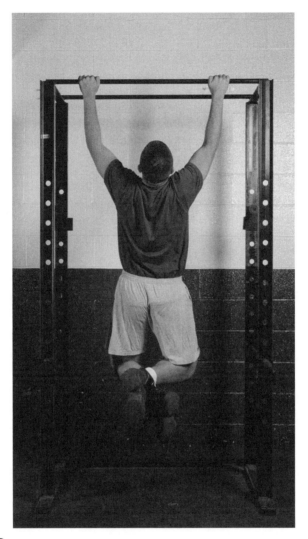

PULL-UPS

There are a variety of different grips used when performing pull-ups which work various groups of arm and back muscles.

REGULAR GRIP

With hands at shoulder width grab the bar with an overhand grip (palms facing away from you) and pull yourself up so your chin is lifted above the bar. Hold yourself above the bar for one second and let yourself down in a slow, controlled manner and repeat.

WIDE GRIP

Performed in the same manner as a regular pull-up with a wider than shoulder width grip.

REVERSE GRIP

With palms facing you grab the bar and pull yourself up so your chin is lifted above the bar. Hold yourself above the bar for one second and let yourself down in a slow, controlled manner and repeat.

CLOSE GRIP

With your hands touching (or within one inch of each other), and palms facing away from you, grab the bar and pull yourself up so your chin is lifted above the bar. Hold yourself above the bar for one second and let yourself down in a slow, controlled manner and repeat.

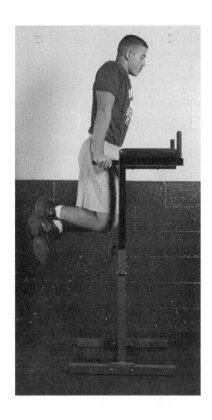 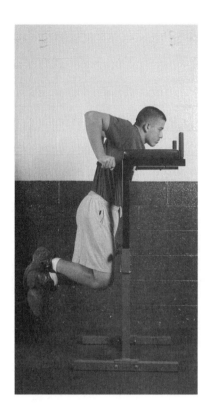

DIPS

Mount two parallel bars with your hands on both sides of your body. Lift your body by straightening your arms. Do not lock your elbows. Slowly lower your body to a level where your arms make a 90-degree angle at the elbow joint. Do not go lower than 90 degrees, because this is bad for your shoulder joints.

Dips train your pectorals, shoulders and triceps.

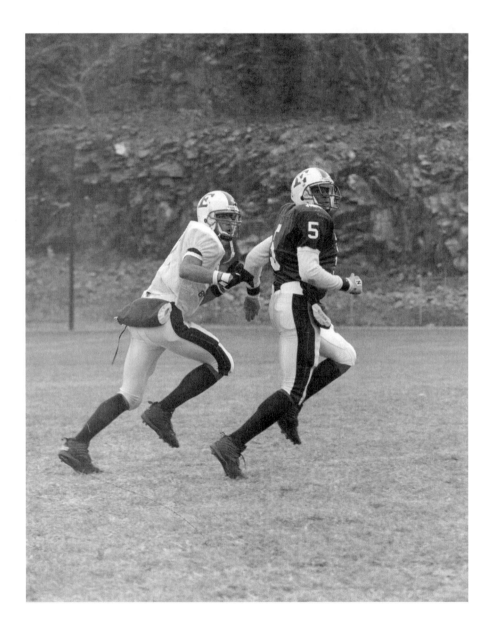

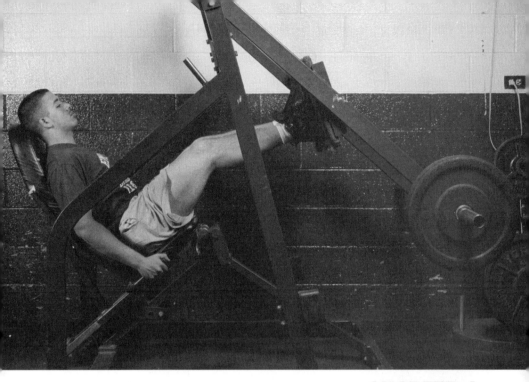

CHAPTER 4:

STRENGTH AND WEIGHT TRAINING

Weight training has become increasingly more important for high school football. In addition to the athletic advantage you hold over your competitor by being bigger, faster and stronger your chances of injury are greatly reduced and your confidence runs higher.

In this book we have attempted to list the most important and popular weight training movements. It is important to keep in mind that equipment can vary greatly between training facilities. While free weights (barbells and dumbbells) are still the preferred method for building stronger, leaner muscle many gyms and coaches have switched to machines such as Nautilus, Cybex, or Hammer. You should consult your coach and determine which type of equipment you prefer.

Just as there are many machines that can take the place of free weights, there are many variations of exercises that can be performed. While reading through the exercises please be aware that many of the exercises can be performed in exactly the same manner using dumbbells or in an alternating fashion. By using dumbbells and/or alternating the movements you are able to further isolate the muscle being trained.

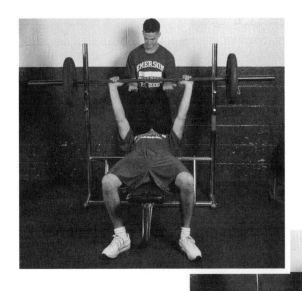

BENCH PRESS

The bench press is a fundamental compound exercise for the upper body and builds the pectorals, deltoids and triceps.

Lie on a flat bench, feet flat on the floor for balance. Grip the bar with a medium grip, and then lift the bar off the rack and hold it at arms length above you. Lower the bar slowly and under control until it touches just above your sternum. The bar should come to a complete stop. Press the bar upward until your arms are fully locked out. Repeat these steps. When set is complete place bar back on rack. Always go through a full range of motion.

Dumbbell bench presses may be done in exactly the same manner as described above, however you will pick up dumbbells from the floor and place them back down on the floor when complete.

Dumbbells will prove to be a bit more difficult to control and you should not attempt to handle the same weight as a barbell bench press.

The incline bench press changes the angle of the movement and applies more stress to the upper chest and deltoids. You will find you cannot handle as much as you can when performing a flat bench press. Incline bench presses, both barbell and dumbbell, are executed exactly the same as bench presses except now you will be on an incline bench. The angle of the incline may vary from bench to bench and can sometimes be changed. As long as the angle is between 0 and 90 degrees you will be training the chest.

Some gyms may also have a decline bench available. By changing the angle, stress is placed on the lower portion of the pectorals and the exercise is performed in precisely the same manner as flat bench and incline bench presses.

Bench presses are the core movement for upper body strength, but a good combination of incline and decline presses along with dumbbell moves will provide you with very well balanced upper body strength.

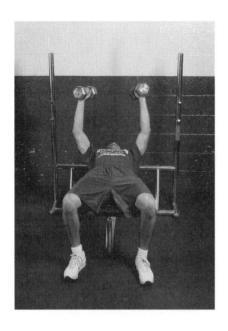 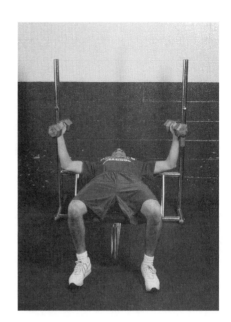

DUMBBELL FLYS

Lie on a bench holding dumbbells at arm's length above you, palms facing one another. Lower the weights out and down to either side in a wide arc as far as you can. Arms may be bent slightly during the movement to reduce stress on the elbows. Bring the weights to a complete stop and lift them back along the same arc (as if giving a hug), the entire time palms facing each other.

Movement may also be performed on incline and decline benches. Additionally there are various machines such as a Pec Deck that will accomplish the same goal as a Fly.

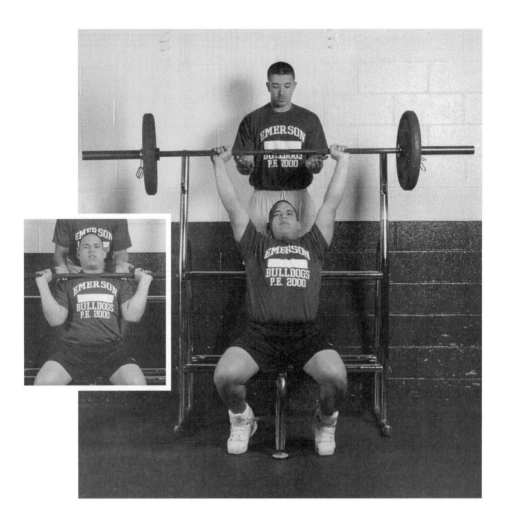

MILITARY PRESS

Military Press is the fundamental movement for shoulder strength and development. From a sitting or standing position grasp the bar with an overhand grip a bit wider than shoulder width apart. Remove bar from the rack and hold weight overhead with arms locked out. Slowly lower the weight down to a position about even with the collarbone. Lift the bar straight up overhead until your arms are locked out. Repeat. When set is completed place bar back on rack.

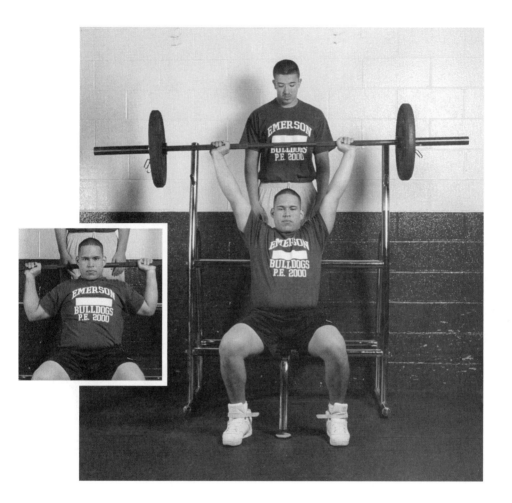

BEHIND THE NECK PRESS

The Behind the Neck Press is executed in the same manner as the military press but the bar is lowered behind your head to the point where the bar touches the trapezious muscles.

Both movements may be performed with dumbbells and can be done in an alternating manner.

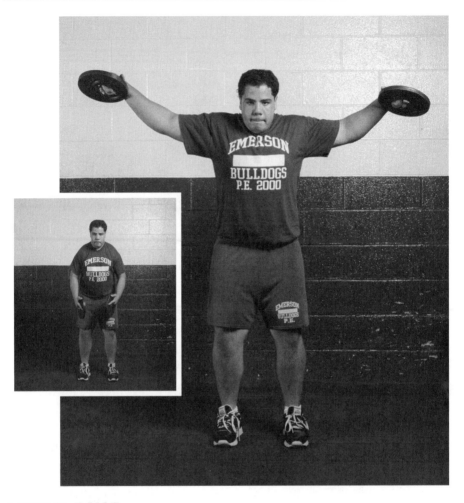

LATERAL RAISE

Take a dumbbell or a plate in each hand and bend forward slightly while bringing the weights together in front of you at arm's length. Lift the weights out and up to either side, turning your wrists slightly as if you were pouring a glass of iced tea. Lift the weights slowly to a point slightly higher than your shoulders, then lower them slowly back down to the starting position.

You may have a tendency to swing or cheat while performing this exercise standing. This can be eliminated by performing the movement while seated at the end of a bench.

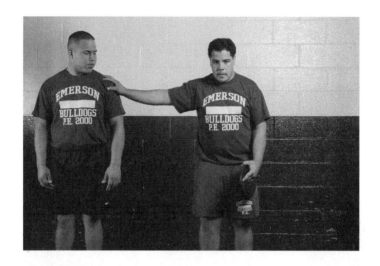

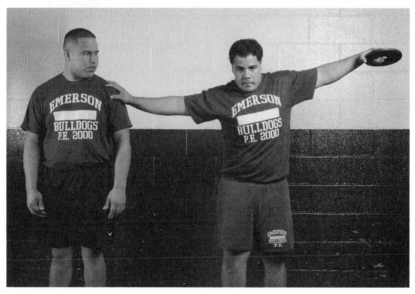

ALTERNATING ONE-ARM LATERAL RAISE

Lateral Raises can also be performed on various machines, with cables and in an alternating manner.

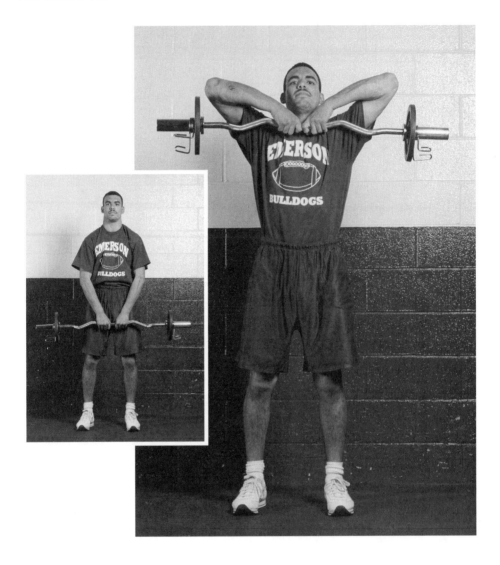

UPRIGHT ROWS

Grasp barbell with an overhand grip and your hands about 6-10 inches apart. Remove bar from rack, or lift bar from the floor, allowing it to hang straight down in front of you. Lift the bar straight up, close to your body to a point just under your chin. From this position lower the bar slowly to the starting position and repeat.

Upright rows may also be performed as Cable Upright Rows with a shorter bar and can be varied with a wider/narrower grip.

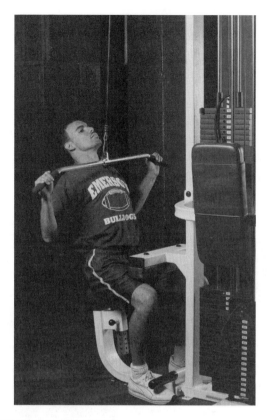

LAT MACHINE PULL DOWNS

This movement can be performed with a variety of bars (wide, close, medium) and grips (overhand, underhand, palms in) and can be executed to the front (chest) or rear (neck). Each bar and grip trains the latimus dorsi muscles at a slightly different angle. It's best to vary bars, grip and type of pull down to receive the best results.

All of the movements are executed in the same manner. Sit on the seat and place knees under pads. Reach up and grasp the bar grip of your choice. Slowly and smoothly pull the weight down to either your upper chest area or trapezius area trying to touch your elbows together behind your back. Pause at the bottom and slowly return the weight to the starting position.

It is vital not to cheat by swinging or pulling the weight violently during these movements or emphasis will be placed on another muscle group.

Lat Machine Pull downs can be substituted with Pull Ups for those who can pull their own body weight up in a strict manner.

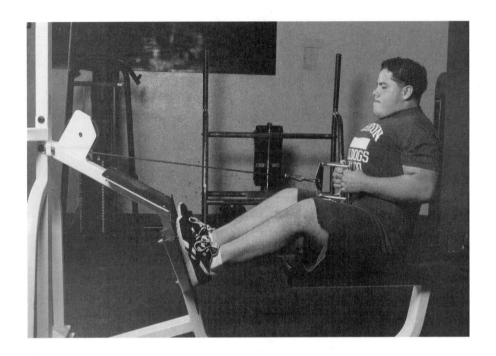

LOW PULLY ROWS

Rowing Movements (Bent Over Row, T-Bar Rows, One Arm Dumbbell Rows):

Rowing movements may be done with a variety of bars and grips or on different machines. All the movements train the muscles of the upper back.

Standing with your feet about shoulder width apart grasp the bar with an overhand or underhand grip. With knees bent slightly, bend forward until your upper body is about parallel to the floor. Keep your back straight and let the bar hang at arm's length below you. Lift the bar upward until it touches the abdominal area and lower it to the starting position, then immediately start your next repetition. A variation of this move may be performed with a T-Bar which stresses a slightly different angle.

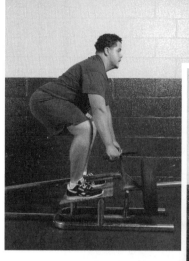

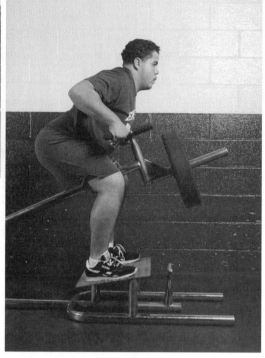

For variation you may choose to perform a One Arm Dumbbell Row. This is performed with one arm at a time while you are supported with a knee on a bench. Follow the same instructions as above with dumbbell.

Some gyms may also have Seated Rowing Machines or Low Pully Row Machines. The fundamental move is executed exactly as a bent over row, however you will be seated with feet supported in front of you.

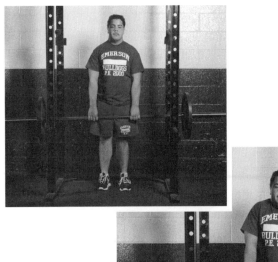

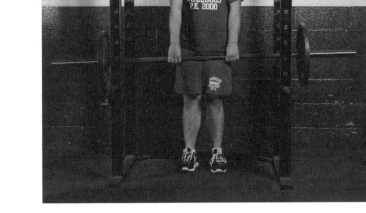

SHRUGS

Stand upright holding barbell or dumbbells at arm's length with an overhand grip. Slowly raise your shoulders as high as you can, as if trying to touch them to your ears. Hold and squeeze for a moment at the top, then lower back down to the starting position and repeat.

Dumbbell shrugs may be done in a seated manner for greater isolation, and shrugs may be performed on a cable system or machine designed specifically for trapezius development.

Because of the nature of the contact in football (a high degree involving the head and neck), major emphasis should be placed on neck development.

HYPER EXTENSIONS

While it is very important to train the muscles of the upper back, the lower back should not be ignored.

Hyper Extensions train the lower back thoroughly. There are specific benches designed for hyper extensions and these can be thought of as a reverse sit-up.

Position yourself face down across a hyper extension bench with your heels hooked under the ankle supports and your hips supported by the pad. Clasp your hands behind your neck and bend forward and down as far as possible, feeling the lower back stretch. From this position raise yourself up to a position just above parallel.

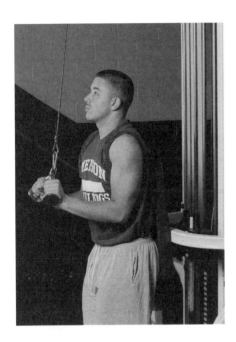 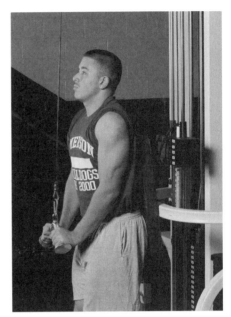

TRICEPS PRESS DOWN

Triceps Press Downs may be performed with a variety of different bars (straight, V, ropes) and are performed on a lat pull down machine.

Stand facing the bar and grasp with an overhand grip about shoulder high. Keep your elbows tucked in at your sides and stationary. Keeping your whole body steady and not leaning, slowly press the bar down as far as possible towards your thighs and lock out your arms feeling the triceps contract. Release and let the bar rise to the starting position and repeat.

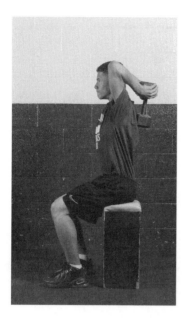 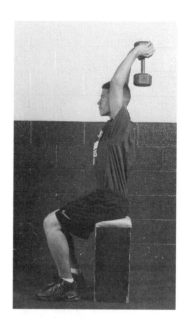

TRICEPS EXTENSIONS/PRESSES

Grasp a dumbbell or barbell, hands close together. Sit on a bench and raise the bar/dumbbell straight up overhead, arms locked out. Keeping your elbows stationary and close to your head, lower the weight down in an arc behind your head until your triceps are fully stretched. Only the forearms move.   From this position press the weight back up overhead to full extension. Lock your arms out and squeeze triceps. Repeat movement.

There have been specific machines designed to perform triceps presses in a stricter manner while seated.

Additionally, you may choose to perform Close Grip Bench Presses (just bring your grip to 6-12 inches apart and perform a bench press) or Half Dips to train your Triceps.

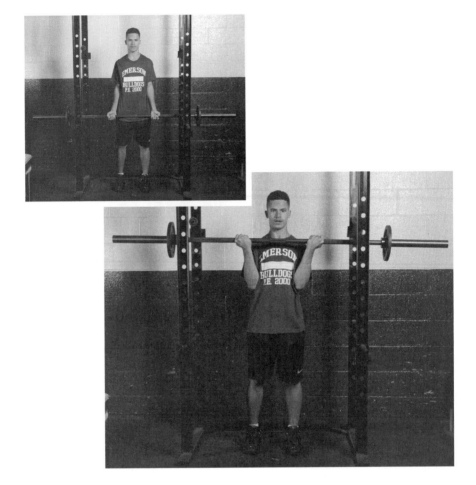

BARBELL CURLS

Stand with feet about shoulder width apart. Grasp the bar with an underhand grip and let it hang at full arm's length in front of you. Curl the bar out and up in a wide arc while keeping your elbows tight to your body. The bar should finish just under your chin. In the same arc slowly lower the bar to the starting position. It is vital not to cheat by swaying, rocking or throwing the weight.

Barbell curls can be done using wide, narrow and moderate grips and will train the biceps at different angles.

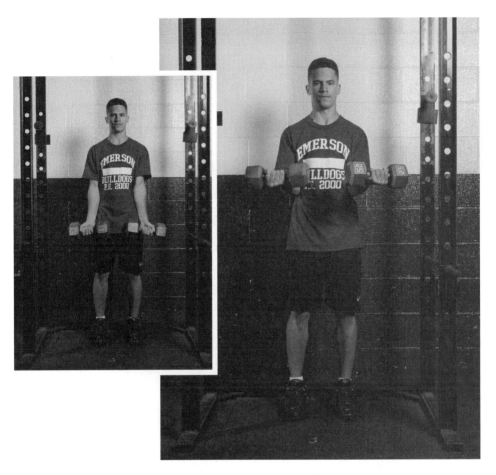

DUMBBELL CURLS

Dumbbell Curls are executed exactly like barbell curls, except you will be grasping dumbbells.

You can vary this movement quite a bit. You may perform dumb-bell curls seated on the end of a bench or on an incline bench. And you can alternate between arms for greater concentration. The biceps will be effectively trained in any of these positions. What you choose should have everything to do with comfort and isolating the muscle.

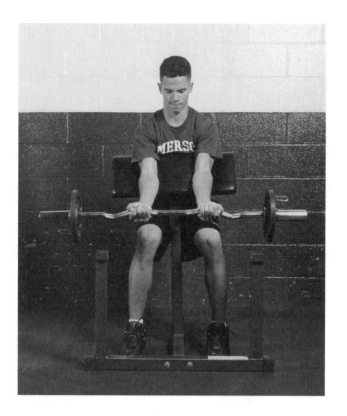

PREACHER CURLS

Preacher Curls utilize a specifically designed bench to completely isolate and help build the biceps.

Start by sitting in the bench. Your arms should be draped over the padding with elbows resting comfortably. Reach forward and grasp the bar with an underhand grip and proceed with a curl.

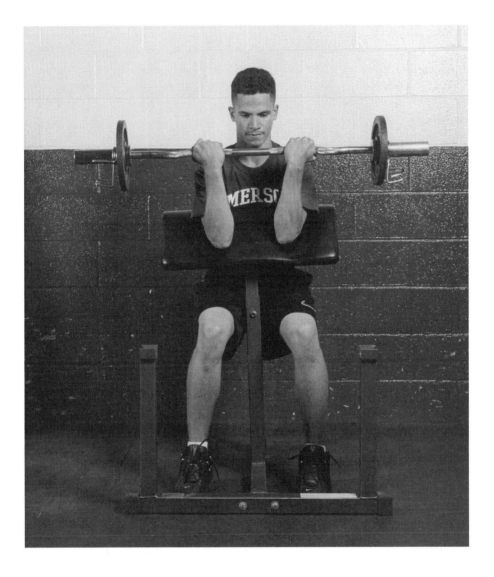

While it is a shorter movement you should feel the total isolation of the biceps. As with many exercises you may vary the grip slightly to train the muscle at a different angle.

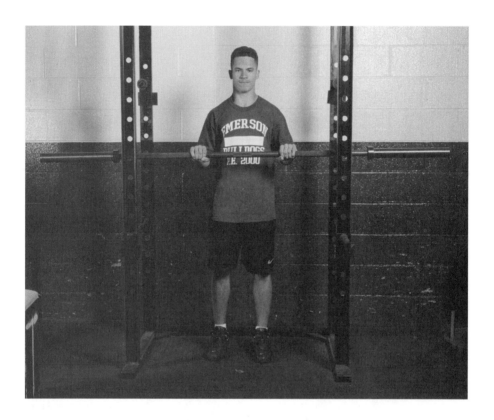

REVERSE CURLS

Reverse Curls are performed in exactly the same manner as a barbell curl, with an overhand grip. Reverse Curls will effectively train the muscles of the forearm and outside edge of the biceps.

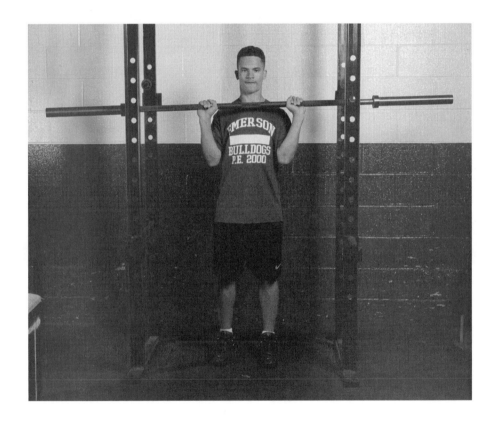

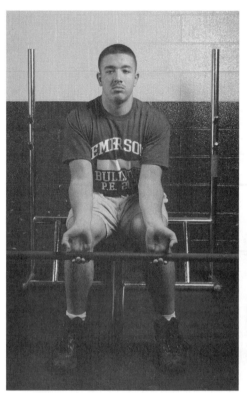 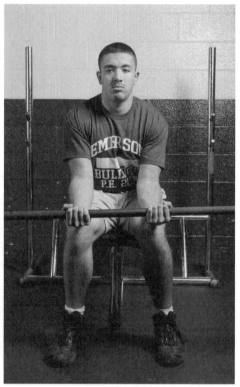

WRIST CURLS

Sit on the edge of a bench and grasp barbell with an underhand grip. Have your forearms resting on your thighs while your hands are hanging over your knees. Keeping every part of your body still, curl your wrist up in an arc from the hanging position so that you can now see your knuckles.

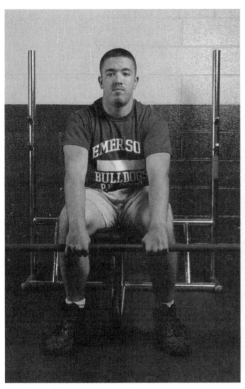 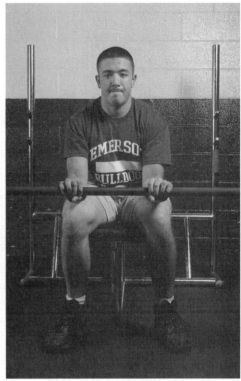

REVERSE WRIST CURLS

Reverse Wrist Curls are executed exactly the same way using an overhand grip.

While the muscles of the forearm are not very large they play an important role in football (i.e. stance, ball carrying, tackling) and should be trained properly.

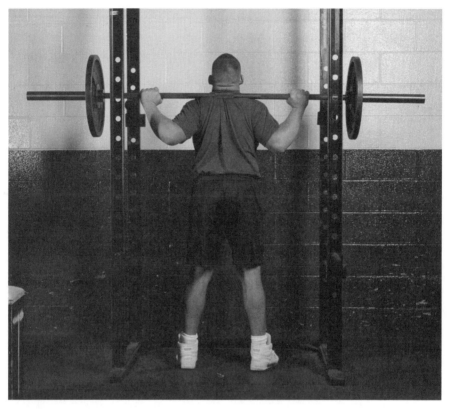

SQUATS

Squats are the fundamental mass and strength building exercise for the lower body, and a key proponent in football success.

With the barbell on a rack, step under it so the bar rests low across the back of your shoulders. Grasp the bar wider than shoulder width for balance, raise up and step away from the rack. Keep your head up and back straight while bending your knees until your thighs are just lower than parallel to the floor. From this point push the weight up to the starting position. To learn the proper technique for squatting a chair or block may be placed under the squatter. The squatter will then be encouraged to sit on the chair or block as a training aid.

A variety of machines have been developed recently that simulate a squat and train the legs at various angles. Additionally you can train your legs at different angles by adjusting your stance.

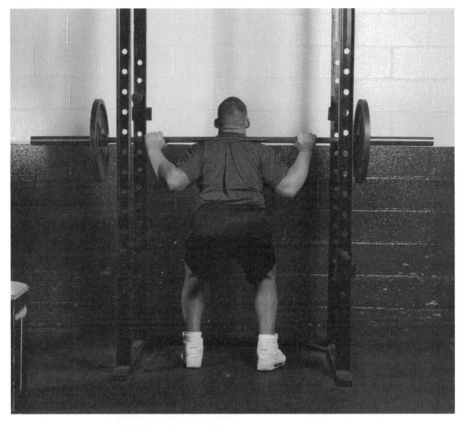

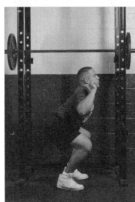

Side view demonstrates proper back arch.

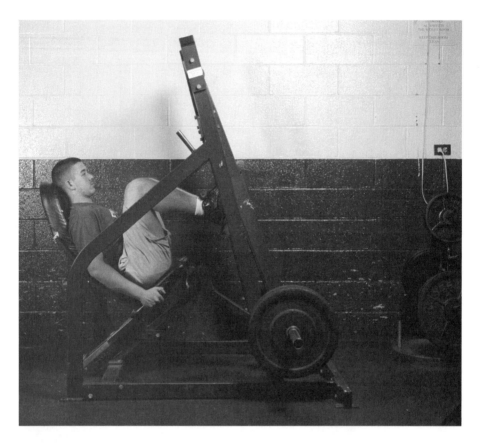

LEG PRESS

There are a variety of Leg Press machines available today. We will refer to the 45-degree leg press in this book. All leg press machines will be used in a similar way.

Position yourself under the machine and place your feet against the crosspiece. Release the safety mechanism and slowly lower the weight by bending your knees into your chest. Bring your knees as close to your chest as possible and push weight up to starting position.

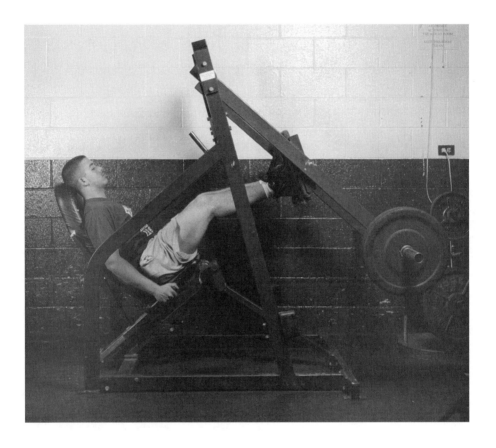

You may vary the move by adjusting your foot position from wide to narrow to toes in and toes out.

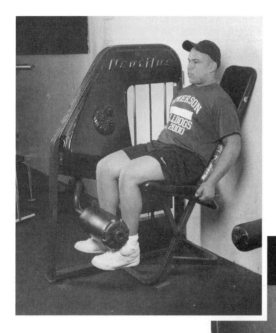

LEG EXTENSIONS

Sit in the seat and hook your feet under the pads. Extend your legs out until your knees are locked out, and squeeze. Lower the weight slowly back to the starting position.

Be sure your buttocks remain on the seat at all times and your back is supported. You may also alternate between legs.

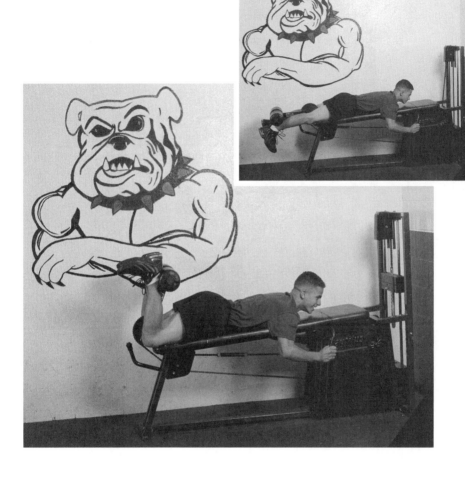

LEG CURLS

Lie face down on the leg curl machine and hook your heels under the pad. Remaining flat on the bench curl your legs up towards your buttocks as far as possible and squeeze. Slowly lower the weight back to the starting position.

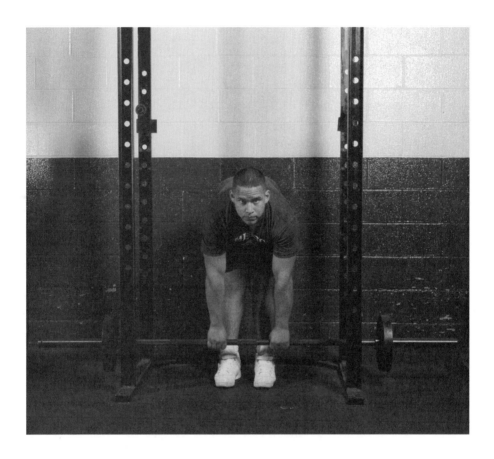

STIFF LEG DEAD LIFTS

Grasp bar with shoulder-width grip and remove from the rack. Keeping your legs locked out, bend forward at the waist, back straight, until your torso is about parallel to the floor, the bar hanging at arm's length below you. Rise to the standing position, pull your shoulders back and arch your spine. Slowly repeat the movement.

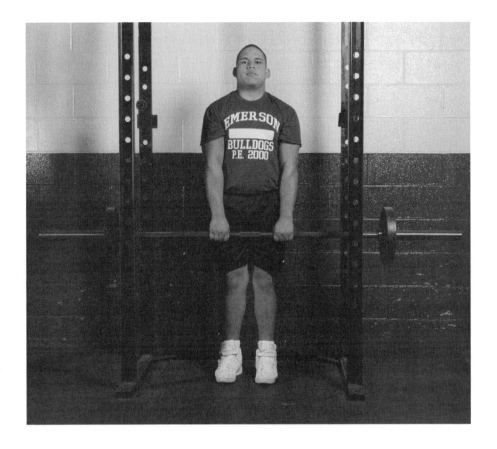

This exercise should be performed with the strictest form to avoid injury or strain.

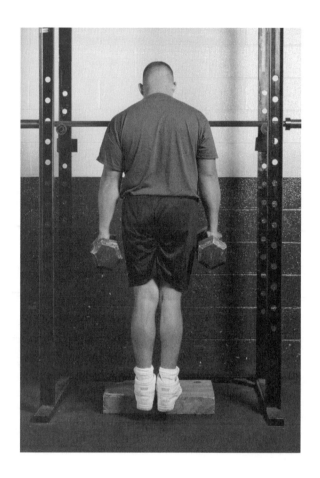

CALF RAISES

Calf raises may be performed with a barbell, dumbbell or on a machine. They may also be done seated and alternating.

The general execution is the same regardless of the training mechanism. Simply rise onto your toes and squeeze, then slowly lower towards your heels and stretch the calf muscle.

To train the calves most effectively a block about 2 inches in height can be placed under your toes for maximum calf contraction.

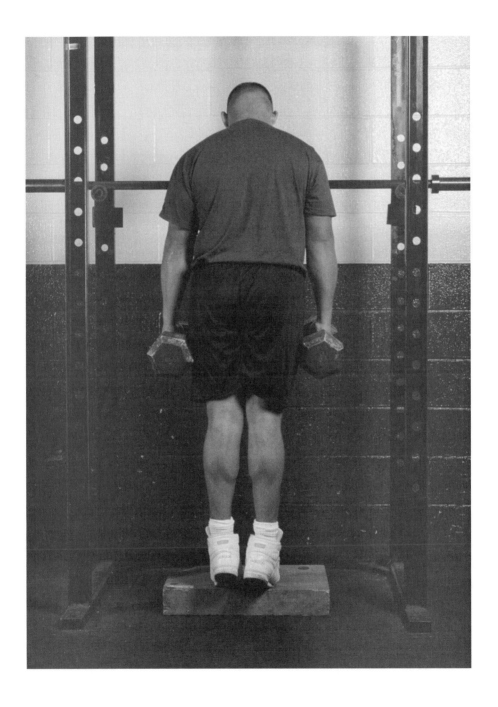

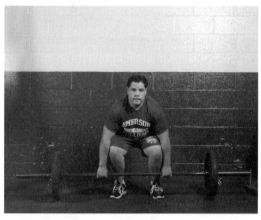

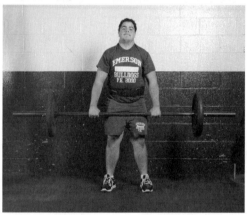

CLEAN AND PRESS

The clean and press builds general body strength and is particularly useful for training for football because the movement is so explosive.

Squat down, lean forward and grasp the bar with an overhand grip about shoulder width apart. Driving with your legs, lift the bar straight up to about shoulder height, then tuck the elbows in and under to support the weight across your upper chest area. Then bend knees slightly, and using the shoulders, arms and legs explosively push the weight overhead.

Reverse the move by slowly bringing the bar back down to your upper chest area. Then bend your knees and reverse the cleaning motion and set the bar back down on the floor.

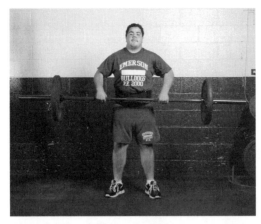

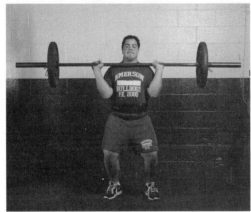

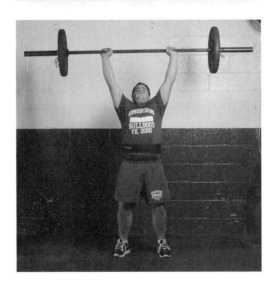

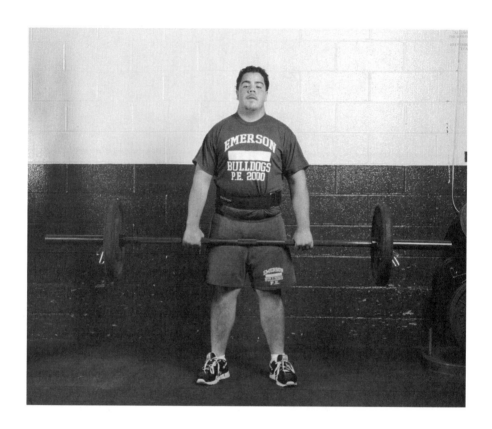

POWER CLEAN

Grasp the bar with an overhand grip about shoulder width apart and let it hang at arm's length in front of you. Bend your knees slightly and drive with your legs. Lift the bar straight up to about shoulder height, then tuck the elbows in and under to support the weight across your upper chest area.

Reverse the cleaning motion and bring bar down to starting position with weight hanging at arm's length.

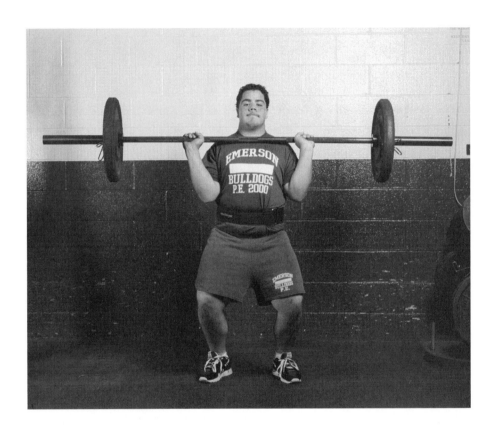

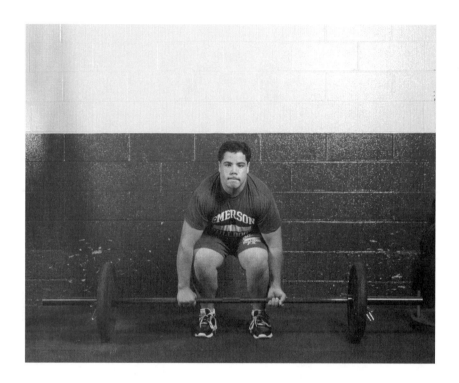

DEAD LIFT

Squat down, lean forward and grasp the bar one hand with an overhand grip and one hand with an underhand grip about shoulder width apart. Driving with your legs, lift the bar straight up keeping your arms locked out. Keep the barbell as close to your shins as possible.

Pull your shoulders back and arch your back at the top of the movement and pause, then slowly lower the weight back to the floor. Of all exercises, you should be able to lift the most weight performing this move because it involves and builds so many body parts.

The dead lift may be performed with a narrower than shoulder width stance or an extremely wide open-toed stance. This is a personal preference and will not train the muscles any differently.

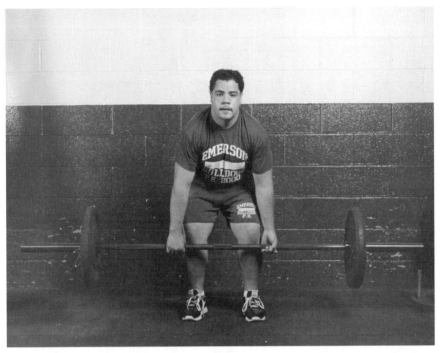

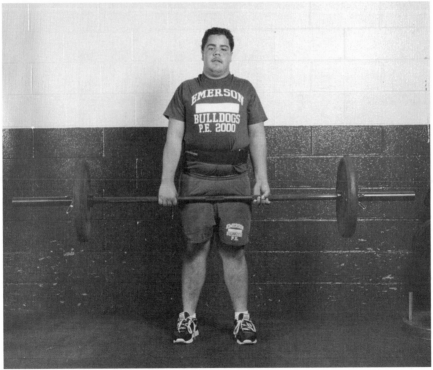

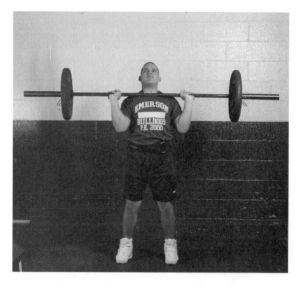

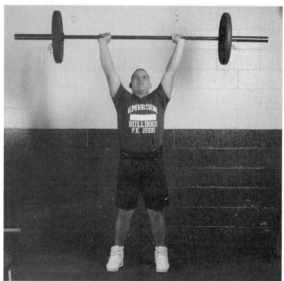

PUSH-PRESS

Grasp the bar in a rack (about shoulder high) with an overhand grip. Lift the bar slightly and step back from the rack. The barbell should be supported across your upper chest by tucking the elbows in and under. Bend knees slightly, and using the shoulders, arms and legs explosively push the weight overhead. Slowly bring the weight down to starting position.

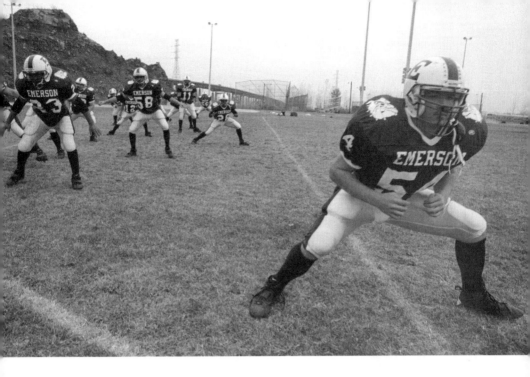

CHAPTER 5:

CONDITIONING

All the weight training in the world will not help you on the football field unless you properly condition your body for the aerobic strain of a football game. Running is a key component of any conditioning program, but simply jogging will not cut it. Rather, a conditioning program should have a balance between stretching, sprinting, distance running, agility and calisthenics.

The idea behind any conditioning program is to prepare the body for the rigors of the activity in which you are partaking. Football requires a balance of cardiovascular fitness and short muscle twitches. By performing specific movements (described in the coming pages) one can attain optimal conditioning levels.

RUNNING

Running sounds simple enough, but it is not! Running plays an important role in every play of a football game; therefore you should pay close attention to your technique when training. As always you should stretch prior to beginning any workout and begin and end each session with a warm up and cool down jog. In addition make sure you are properly equipped for the type of training you are performing (e.g. you may want to wear running sneakers for a distance run, but football cleats for your agility drills).

By far the most important technique of proper running is breathing. The proper breath is a very deep inhalation and exhalation. Deep breaths get more oxygen to your muscles, rid your body of carbon dioxide, and aid in reducing fatigue.

Relaxing the upper body is another important running technique. When you are running the only body parts that should be working are your lungs and your legs. If your upper body, fists, or face are clenched or flexed while running, the blood that should be going to your legs is sent to the flexed body parts as well, thus decreasing the amount of oxygen to your legs. Try to relax and breathe deeply.

A full arm swing will help you get into a good running step and breathing rhythm. Your hands should swing in a straight line from your hips to your chest. Elbows should be bent slightly and hands should be loose and unclenched.

Distance running builds the cardiovascular strength necessary to compete effectively throughout four quarters of a football game. It can be performed on a track or treadmill or simply by running through town. Running up and down hill as well as bleachers or steps can be an interesting and helpful twist to your training.

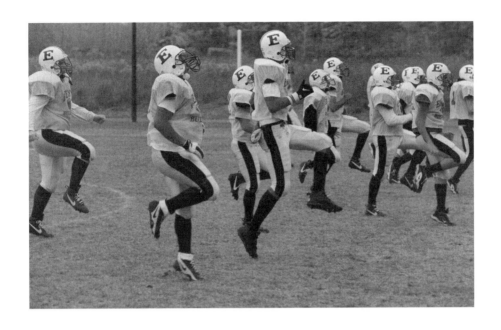

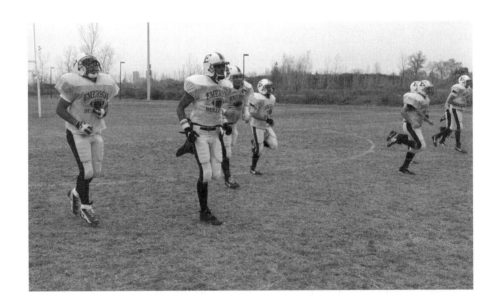

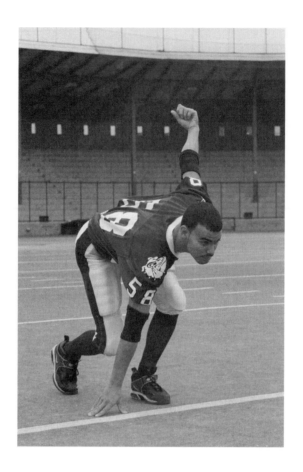

SPRINTING

Sprinting builds the explosiveness needed to start from a set position and perform at maximum effort for the length of the play. Sprinting also builds cardiovascular strength.

Because the actual length and time of a football play varies you should focus on specific distances to prepare yourself for a season. Those distances should be 20 yards, 40 yards, 60 yards, 100 yards and 200 yards. When performing the 100 and 200 yard varieties you should use a football field and run sideline to sideline. This will encourage lateral stability through the transition and acclimate you to the playing surface. You should also begin each sprint from your football stance (by position).

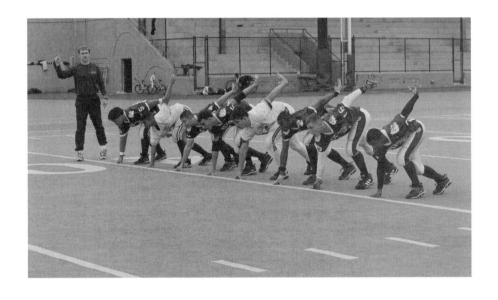

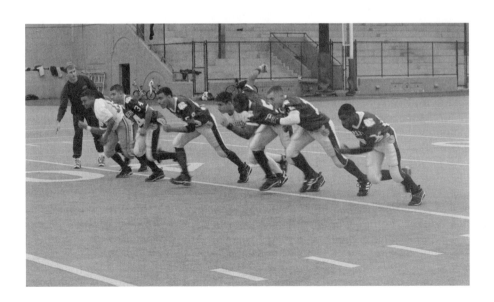

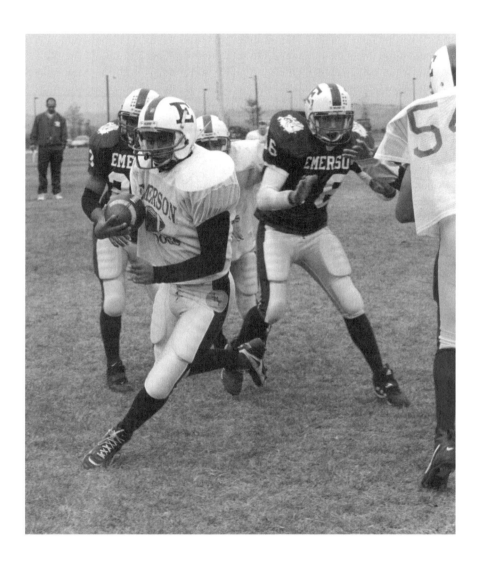

AGILITY DRILLS

Agility drills are a sport specific training technique designed to get the athlete moving faster and more fluidly. Agility drills can range from something as simple as running backwards to a complex network of actions and jumps.

We will focus on the most popular football specific drills that you can perform on your own. Your coach will most likely introduce additional drills during practices, particularly drills that focus on your position. For example, quarterbacks and wide receivers will practice passing and catching drills, while offensive and defensive linemen will practice blocking drills.

In addition, there are a variety of partner drills that you can perform with a workout partner. You'll be introduced to a lot of these exercises, such as wheelbarrows, on the field during practice.

A good way to mix up your workout is to set up station drills. You will most likely perform these during practice as well. Pick four exercises such as jumping jacks, shuttle drills, carriogas, and tires/ropes. (You could also choose any calisthenics exercise or agility drill.) Start at one corner of a square (about 20 yards). Perform the first exercise for 30 seconds, and then quickly sprint to the next corner for the next exercise. Continue until all exercises have been completed. If you begin station drills at the start of your 12-week workout, you should be able to build up to about 2 minutes for each exercise.

SHUTTLES

Shuttles are performed to increase speed and productivity through lateral movements, and increase your foot speed. Start in an athletic position, knees slightly bent, hands hanging athletically at your sides. Begin by moving your left instep laterally towards your right instep. When it arrives shuttle your right foot laterally away from your left foot. Continue down your path in a straight line keeping your head up and body facing in the direction you began. You may choose to stop and reverse direction at certain points. You may feel a burn in your inner thighs as these are muscles not effectively trained by weightlifting, running or sprinting, but play a key role to a football player.

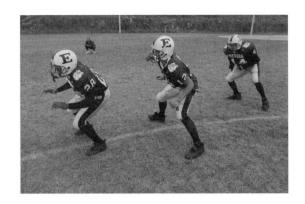

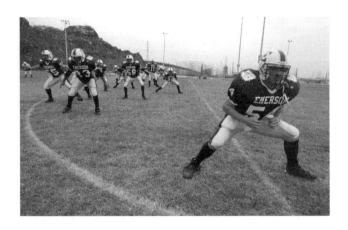

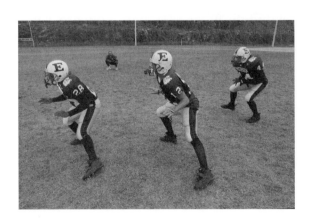

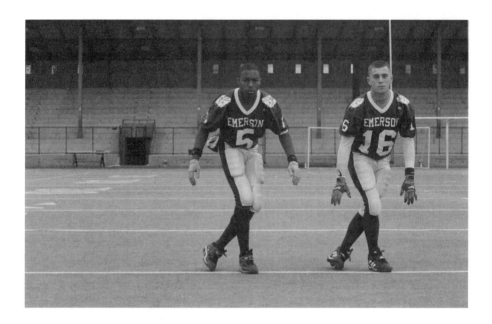

CARRIOGA

Carriogas build foot speed and enhance your coordination. Start in an athletic position, knees slightly bent, hands hanging athletically at your sides, trunk leaning very slightly forward so that your center of gravity is over the balls of your feet. Your shoulders and arms stay aligned with the direction of movement, so that rotation occurs only in your hips and lower back.

Cross your left foot in front of your right foot and plant it by the side of and slightly ahead of your right foot. Cross your right foot behind your left foot and plant it so that your feet are in their normal positions. Cross your left foot behind your right foot and plant it to the side of and slightly behind your right foot. Cross your right foot in front of your left foot so that your feet are back in their normal positions. Repeat these moves.

As you become familiar with the sequence you should focus on speed, explosion and differing patterns.

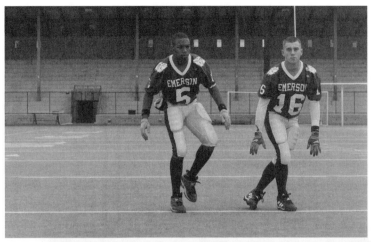

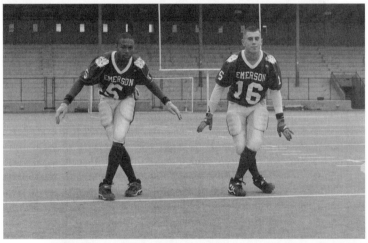

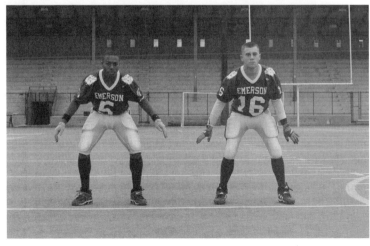

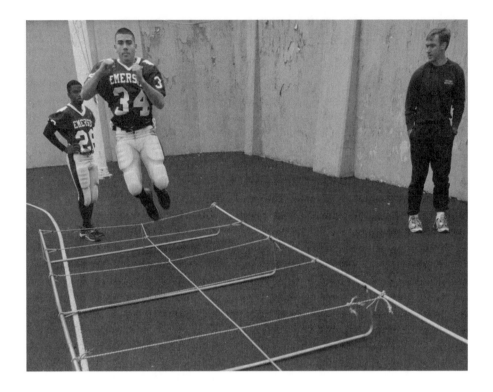

ROPES OR TIRES (GRID):

Rope and Tire Grids are quite versatile and exceptional for speed and agility. You can perform various movements through the grid. You may simply run through the grid with a focus on high knees and explosion. You may hop having one foot land in each box/tire. You can perform alternating hops with feet together. You may choose to perform one-legged hops. There is no wrong way to perform the drill as long as you are pumping your arms and legs.

When you have become particularly agile and confident you may try any of the movements above, laterally. Or for the very daring, Carrioga through the rope/tires.

As you get closer to the season you may combine the ropes/tires with other movements such as a tackling drill or a pass reception. These work on your eye-hand coordination as well as your footwork.

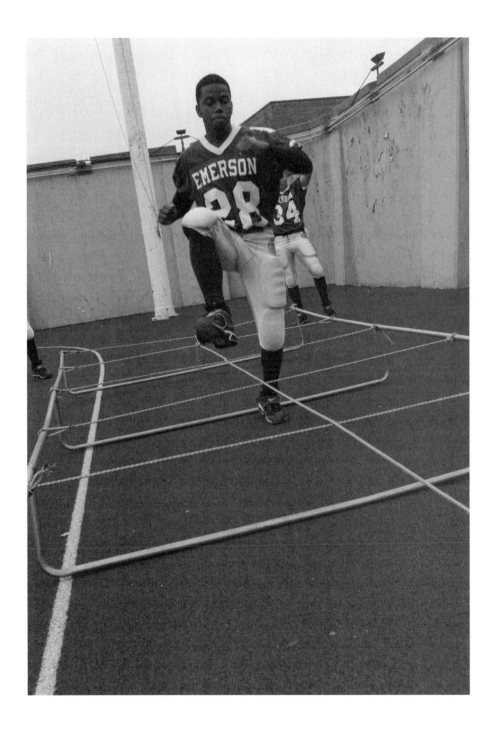

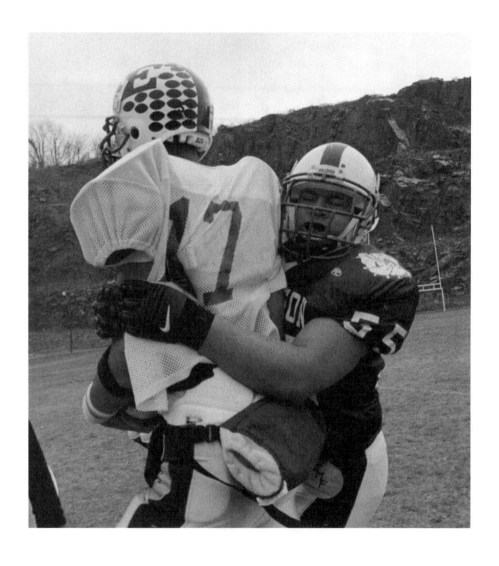

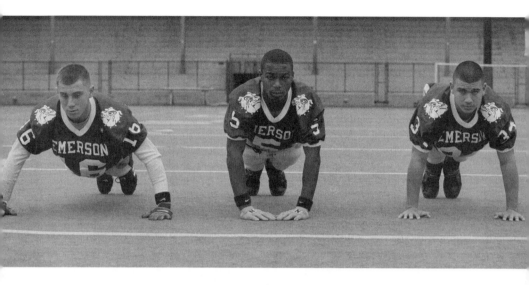

CHAPTER 6:
THE FOOTBALL WORKOUT

This workout is a 12-week workout, divided into three 4-week sections combining weight training and conditioning. It is designed with increasing intensity through each of the three cycles. You should begin and end each session with 10 to 15 minutes of stretching (see Chapter 2).

If you find that the workout is too challenging (or too easy), try beginning at a later point in the 12-week cycle, or repeating a cycle until you are comfortable increasing sets and reps. The amount of weight to be used in each weight training exercise will vary from person to person, but a good rule of thumb is to start at a lower weight and not over-do it. You should consult with your strength coach as to the most appropriate weight for your age and size.

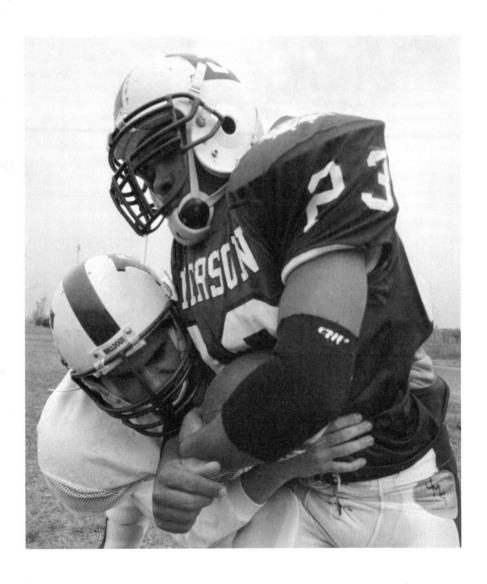

This workout was designed with flexibility in mind. We've designed the workout on a 6-day cycle, rather than assigning a specific day. Therefore, if you skip a day, you can just resume where you left off, or if you find a particular order works better for you, you can swap days (do Day 1 exercises on Day 4 or 5, for example) or combine days to accommodate your schedule (doing Day 1 and 2, for example, on one day, and allowing yourself an extra day off). It is important to maintain your strength program throughout the football season; however, the workout will vary greatly due to the physical demands of football practice. Your coaches will instruct you as to an appropriate strength maintenance program during the season.

As with any workout, consult with your doctor if you have any questions about your health or safety.

WEEK 1

DAY 1

CHEST

Bench Press
1 x warm-up
3 x 12

Incline Bench Press
1 x warm-up
3 x 12

Flys (any variation
including machine)
3 x 12

TRICEPS

Triceps Press-downs
(any grip)
1 x warm-up
3 x 12

Triceps Extensions
1 x warm-up
3 x 12

(You may want to do
the close-grip bench
press for 3 x 12 on this
day as well.)

DAY 2

CONDITIONING

¼ mile warm-up run

AGILITY DRILLS

Shuttles
2 x 40 yards

Carrioga
2 x 40 yards

Ropes/Tires
3 sets

CALISTHENICS

Push-Ups
2 x 25

Abdominal Exercise
(your choice)
3 x 25

SPRINTS

3 X 20 yards
3 X 40 yards
3 X 60 yards

¼ mile cool-down run

DAY 3

LEGS

Squats
2 x warm-up
3 x 12

Leg Press (any variety)
1 x warm-up
3 x 12

Leg Extensions
3 x 12

Leg Curls
3 x 12

Calf Raises
(any variety)
1 x warm-up
3 x 12

BICEPS

Barbell Curls
1 x warm-up
3 x 12

Preacher Curls
1 x warm-up
3 x 12

Forearms
1 x warm-up
3 x 12

Wrist Curls
1 x warm-up
3 x 12

WEEK 1

DAY 4

CONDITIONING

1 ¼ mile distance run

CALISTHENICS

Squats
2 X 20

Walking Lunges
2 X 20 yards

Calf Raises
2 X 25

SPRINTS

2 x 100 yards
2 X 200 yards

¼ mile cool-down run

DAY 5

BACK

Dead Lift
2 x warm-up
3 x 12

Power Clean
1 x warm-up
3 x 12

Bent-over Row
1 x warm-up
3 x 12

Lat Pull-downs
3 x 12

Hyper-extensions
3 x 12

SHOULDERS

Push-press
1 x warm-up
3 x 12

Military Press (or
Behind-the-neck Press)
3 x 12

Lateral Raises
3 x 12

Shrugs
1 x warm-up
3 x 12

DAY 6

CONDITIONING

¼ mile warm-up run

AGILITY DRILLS

Shuttles
2 x 40 yards

Carrioga
2 x 40 yards

Ropes/Tires
3 sets

CALISTHENICS

Push-Ups
2 x 25

Abdominal Exercise
(your choice)
3 x 25

SPRINTS

3 X 20 yards
3 X 40 yards
3 X 60 yards

¼ mile cool-down run

WEEK 2

DAY 1

CHEST

Bench Press
1 x warm-up
3 x 12

Incline Bench Press
1 x warm-up
3 x 12

Flys (any variation
including machine)
3 x 12

TRICEPS

Triceps Press-downs
(any grip)
1 x warm-up
3 x 12

Triceps Extensions
1 x warm-up
3 x 12

(You may want to do
the close-grip bench
press for 3 x 12 on this
day as well.)

DAY 2

CONDITIONING

¼ mile warm-up run

AGILITY DRILLS

Shuttles
2 x 40 yards

Carrioga
2 x 40 yards

Ropes/Tires
3 sets

CALISTHENICS

Push-Ups
2 x 25

Abdominal Exercise
(your choice)
3 x 25

SPRINTS

3 X 20 yards
3 X 40 yards
3 X 60 yards

¼ mile cool-down run

DAY 3

LEGS

Squats
2 x warm-up
3 x 12

Leg Press (any variety)
1 x warm-up
3 x 12

Leg Extensions
3 x 12

Leg Curls
3 x 12

Calf Raises
(any variety)
1 x warm-up
3 x 12

BICEPS

Barbell Curls
1 x warm-up
3 x 12

Preacher Curls
1 x warm-up
3 x 12

Forearms
1 x warm-up
3 x 12

Wrist Curls
1 x warm-up
3 x 12

DAY 4

CONDITIONING

1 ¼ mile distance run

CALISTHENICS

Squats
2 X 20

Walking Lunges
2 X 20 yards

Calf Raises
2 X 25

SPRINTS

2 x 100 yards
2 X 200 yards

¼ mile cool-down run

DAY 5

BACK

Dead Lift
2 x warm-up
3 x 12

Power Clean
1 x warm-up
3 x 12

Bent-over Row
1 x warm-up
3 x 12

Lat Pull-downs
3 x 12

Hyper-extensions
3 x 12

SHOULDERS

Push-press
1 x warm-up
3 x 12

Military Press (or
Behind-the-neck Press)
3 x 12

Lateral Raises
3 x 12

Shrugs
1 x warm-up
3 x 12

DAY 6

CONDITIONING

¼ mile warm-up run

AGILITY DRILLS

Shuttles
2 x 40 yards

Carrioga
2 x 40 yards

Ropes/Tires
3 sets

CALISTHENICS

Push-Ups
2 x 25

Abdominal Exercise
(your choice)
3 x 25

SPRINTS

3 X 20 yards
3 X 40 yards
3 X 60 yards

¼ mile cool-down run

WEEK 3

DAY 1	DAY 2	DAY 3
CHEST	**CONDITIONING**	**LEGS**
Bench Press 1 x warm-up 3 x 12	¼ mile warm-up run	Squats 2 x warm-up 3 x 12
Incline Bench Press 1 x warm-up 3 x 12	**AGILITY DRILLS** Shuttles 2 x 40 yards	Leg Press (any variety) 1 x warm-up 3 x 12
Flys (any variation including machine) 3 x 12	Carrioga 2 x 40 yards	Leg Extensions 3 x 12
TRICEPS	Ropes/Tires 3 sets	Leg Curls 3 x 12
Triceps Press-downs (any grip) 1 x warm-up 3 x 12	**CALISTHENICS** Push-Ups 2 x 25	Calf Raises (any variety) 1 x warm-up 3 x 12
Triceps Extensions 1 x warm-up 3 x 12	Abdominal Exercise (your choice) 3 x 25	**BICEPS**
(You may want to do the close-grip bench press for 3 x 12 on this day as well.)	**SPRINTS** 3 X 20 yards 3 X 40 yards 3 X 60 yards	Barbell Curls 1 x warm-up 3 x 12
		Preacher Curls 1 x warm-up 3 x 12
	¼ mile cool-down run	Forearms 1 x warm-up 3 x 12
		Wrist Curls 1 x warm-up 3 x 12

WEEK 3

DAY 4

CONDITIONING

1 ¼ mile distance run

CALISTHENICS

Squats
2 X 20

Walking Lunges
2 X 20 yards

Calf Raises
2 X 25

SPRINTS

2 x 100 yards
2 X 200 yards

¼ mile cool-down run

DAY 5

BACK

Dead Lift
2 x warm-up
3 x 12

Power Clean
1 x warm-up
3 x 12

Bent-over Row
1 x warm-up
3 x 12

Lat Pull-downs
3 x 12

Hyper-extensions
3 x 12

SHOULDERS

Push-press
1 x warm-up
3 x 12

Military Press (or
Behind-the-neck Press)
3 x 12

Lateral Raises
3 x 12

Shrugs
1 x warm-up
3 x 12

DAY 6

CONDITIONING

¼ mile warm-up run

AGILITY DRILLS

Shuttles
2 x 40 yards

Carrioga
2 x 40 yards

Ropes/Tires
3 sets

CALISTHENICS

Push-Ups
2 x 25

Abdominal Exercise
(your choice)
3 x 25

SPRINTS

3 X 20 yards
3 X 40 yards
3 X 60 yards

¼ mile cool-down run

WEEK 4

DAY 1

CHEST

Bench Press
1 x warm-up
3 x 12

Incline Bench Press
1 x warm-up
3 x 12

Flys (any variation
including machine)
3 x 12

TRICEPS

Triceps Press-downs
(any grip)
1 x warm-up
3 x 12

Triceps Extensions
1 x warm-up
3 x 12

(You may want to do
the close-grip bench
press for 3 x 12 on this
day as well.)

DAY 2

CONDITIONING

¼ mile warm-up run

AGILITY DRILLS

Shuttles
2 x 40 yards

Carrioga
2 x 40 yards

Ropes/Tires
3 sets

CALISTHENICS

Push-Ups
2 x 25

Abdominal Exercise
(your choice)
3 x 25

SPRINTS

3 X 20 yards
3 X 40 yards
3 X 60 yards

¼ mile cool-down run

DAY 3

LEGS

Squats
2 x warm-up
3 x 12

Leg Press (any variety)
1 x warm-up
3 x 12

Leg Extensions
3 x 12

Leg Curls
3 x 12

Calf Raises
(any variety)
1 x warm-up
3 x 12

BICEPS

Barbell Curls
1 x warm-up
3 x 12

Preacher Curls
1 x warm-up
3 x 12

Forearms
1 x warm-up
3 x 12

Wrist Curls
1 x warm-up
3 x 12

DAY 4

CONDITIONING

1 ¼ mile distance run

CALISTHENICS

Squats
2 X 20

Walking Lunges
2 X 20 yards

Calf Raises
2 X 25

SPRINTS

2 x 100 yards
2 X 200 yards

¼ mile cool-down run

DAY 5

BACK

Dead Lift
2 x warm-up
3 x 12

Power Clean
1 x warm-up
3 x 12

Bent-over Row
1 x warm-up
3 x 12

Lat Pull-downs
3 x 12

Hyper-extensions
3 x 12

SHOULDERS

Push-press
1 x warm-up
3 x 12

Military Press (or
Behind-the-neck Press)
3 x 12

Lateral Raises
3 x 12

Shrugs
1 x warm-up
3 x 12

DAY 6

CONDITIONING

¼ mile warm-up run

Agility drills
Shuttles
2 x 40 yards

Carrioga
2 x 40 yards

Ropes/Tires
3 sets

CALISTHENICS

Push-Ups
2 x 25

Abdominal Exercise
(your choice)
3 x 25

SPRINTS

3 X 20 yards
3 X 40 yards
3 X 60 yards

¼ mile cool-down run

WEEK 5

DAY 1

CHEST

Bench Press
1 x warm-up
4 x 8

Incline Bench Press
1 x warm-up
4 x 8

Flys (any variation
including machine)
4 x 8

Dumbbell Bench Press
(any variety)
4 x 8

TRICEPS

Triceps Press-downs
(any grip)
1 x warm-up
4 x 8

Triceps Extensions
1 x warm-up
4 x 8

Close Grip Bench
4 x 8

DAY 2

CONDITIONING

½ mile warm-up run

AGILITY DRILLS

Shuttles
3 x 40 yards

Carrioga
3 x 40 yards

Ropes/Tires
3 sets

CALISTHENICS

Push-Ups
3 x 25

Abdominal Exercise
(your choice)
3 x 25

SPRINTS

4 X 20 yards
4 X 40 yards
4 X 60 yards

½ mile cool-down run

DAY 3

LEGS

Squats
2 x warm-up
4 x 8

Leg Press (any variety)
1 x warm-up
4 x 8

Leg Extensions
4 x 8

Leg Curls
4 x 8

Calf Raises
(any variety)
1 x warm-up
4 x 8

BICEPS

Barbell Curls
1 x warm-up
4 x 8

Preacher Curls
1 x warm-up
4 x 8

Dumbbell Curls
(any variety)
4 x 8

Forearms
1 x warm-up
3 x 12

Wrist Curls
1 x warm-up
3 x 12

DAY 4

CONDITIONING

2 mile distance run

CALISTHENICS

Squats
2 X 20

Walking Lunges
2 X 20 yards

Calf Raises
2 X 25

SPRINTS

3 x 100 yards
3 X 200 yards

½ mile cool-down run

DAY 5

BACK

Dead Lift
2 x warm-up
4 x 8

Power Clean
1 x warm-up
4 x 8

Bent-over Row
1 x warm-up
4 x 8

Lat Pull-downs
4 x 8

Hyper-extensions
4 x 8

SHOULDERS

Push-press
1 x warm-up
4 x 8

Military Press (or
Behind-the-neck Press)
4 x 8

Lateral Raises
4 x 8

Shrugs
1 x warm-up
4 x 8

Upright Rows
4 x 8

DAY 6

CONDITIONING

½ mile warm-up run

AGILITY DRILLS

Shuttles
3 x 40 yards

Carrioga
3 x 40 yards

Ropes/Tires
3 sets

CALISTHENICS

Push-Ups
3 x 25

Abdominal Exercise
(your choice)
3 x 25

SPRINTS

4 X 20 yards
4 X 40 yards
4 X 60 yards

½ mile cool-down run

WEEK 6

DAY 1

CHEST

Bench Press
1 x warm-up
4 x 8

Incline Bench Press
1 x warm-up
4 x 8

Flys (any variation
including machine)
4 x 8

Dumbbell Bench Press
(any variety)
4 x 8

TRICEPS

Triceps Press-downs
(any grip)
1 x warm-up
4 x 8

Triceps Extensions
1 x warm-up
4 x 8

Close Grip Bench
4 x 8

DAY 2

CONDITIONING

½ mile warm-up run

AGILITY DRILLS

Shuttles
3 x 40 yards

Carrioga
3 x 40 yards

Ropes/Tires
3 sets

CALISTHENICS

Push-Ups
3 x 25

Abdominal Exercise
(your choice)
3 x 25

SPRINTS

4 X 20 yards
4 X 40 yards
4 X 60 yards

½ mile cool-down run

DAY 3

LEGS

Squats
2 x warm-up
4 x 8

Leg Press (any variety)
1 x warm-up
4 x 8

Leg Extensions
4 x 8

Leg Curls
4 x 8

Calf Raises
(any variety)
1 x warm-up
4 x 8

BICEPS

Barbell Curls
1 x warm-up
4 x 8

Preacher Curls
1 x warm-up
4 x 8

Dumbbell Curls
(any variety)
4 x 8

Forearms
1 x warm-up
3 x 12

Wrist Curls
1 x warm-up
3 x 12

DAY 4

CONDITIONING

2 mile distance run

CALISTHENICS

Squats
2 X 20

Walking Lunges
2 X 20 yards

Calf Raises
2 X 25

SPRINTS

3 x 100 yards
3 X 200 yards

½ mile cool-down run

DAY 5

BACK

Dead Lift
2 x warm-up
4 x 8

Power Clean
1 x warm-up
4 x 8

Bent-over Row
1 x warm-up
4 x 8

Lat Pull-downs
4 x 8

Hyper-extensions
4 x 8

SHOULDERS

Push-press
1 x warm-up
4 x 8

Military Press (or
Behind-the-neck Press)
4 x 8

Lateral Raises
4 x 8

Shrugs
1 x warm-up
4 x 8

Upright Rows
4 x 8

DAY 6

CONDITIONING

½ mile warm-up run

AGILITY DRILLS

Shuttles
3 x 40 yards

Carrioga
3 x 40 yards

Ropes/Tires
3 sets

CALISTHENICS

Push-Ups
3 x 25

Abdominal Exercise
(your choice)
3 x 25

SPRINTS

4 X 20 yards
4 X 40 yards
4 X 60 yards

½ mile cool-down run

WEEK 7

DAY 1

CHEST

Bench Press
1 x warm-up
4 x 8

Incline Bench Press
1 x warm-up
4 x 8

Flys (any variation
including machine)
4 x 8

Dumbbell Bench Press
(any variety)
4 x 8

TRICEPS

Triceps Press-downs
(any grip)
1 x warm-up
4 x 8

Triceps Extensions
1 x warm-up
4 x 8

Close Grip Bench
4 x 8

DAY 2

CONDITIONING

½ mile warm-up run

AGILITY DRILLS

Shuttles
3 x 40 yards

Carrioga
3 x 40 yards

Ropes/Tires
3 sets

CALISTHENICS

Push-Ups
3 x 25

Abdominal Exercise
(your choice)
3 x 25

SPRINTS

4 X 20 yard
4 X 40 yards
4 X 60 yards

½ mile cool-down run

DAY 3

LEGS

Squats
2 x warm-up
4 x 8

Leg Press (any variety)
1 x warm-up
4 x 8

Leg Extensions
4 x 8

Leg Curls
4 x 8

Calf Raises
(any variety)
1 x warm-up
4 x 8

BICEPS

Barbell Curls
1 x warm-up
4 x 8

Preacher Curls
1 x warm-up
4 x 8

Dumbbell Curls
(any variety)
4 x 8

Forearms
1 x warm-up
3 x 12

Wrist Curls
1 x warm-up
3 x 12

DAY 4

CONDITIONING

2 mile distance run

CALISTHENICS

Squats
2 X 20

Walking Lunges
2 X 20 yards

Calf Raises
2 X 25

SPRINTS

3 x 100 yards
3 X 200 yards

½ mile cool-down run

DAY 5

BACK

Dead Lift
2 x warm-up
4 x 8

Power Clean
1 x warm-up
4 x 8

Bent-over Row
1 x warm-up
4 x 8

Lat Pull-downs
4 x 8

Hyper-extensions
4 x 8

SHOULDERS

Push-press
1 x warm-up
4 x 8

Military Press (or
Behind-the-neck Press)
4 x 8

Lateral Raises
4 x 8

Shrugs
1 x warm-up
4 x 8

Upright Rows
4 x 8

DAY 6

CONDITIONING

½ mile warm-up run

AGILITY DRILLS

Shuttles
3 x 40 yards

Carrioga
3 x 40 yards

Ropes/Tires
3 sets

CALISTHENICS

Push-Ups
3 x 25

Abdominal Exercise
(your choice)
3 x 25

SPRINTS

4 X 20 yards
4 X 40 yards
4 X 60 yards

½ mile cool-down run

WEEK 8

DAY 1	DAY 2	DAY 3

DAY 1

CHEST

Bench Press
1 x warm-up
4 x 8

Incline Bench Press
1 x warm-up
4 x 8

Flys (any variation
including machine)
4 x 8

Dumbbell Bench Press
(any variety)
4 x 8

TRICEPS

Triceps Press-downs
(any grip)
1 x warm-up
4 x 8

Triceps Extensions
1 x warm-up
4 x 8

Close Grip Bench
4 x 8

DAY 2

CONDITIONING

½ mile warm-up run

AGILITY DRILLS

Shuttles
3 x 40 yards

Carrioga
3 x 40 yards

Ropes/Tires
3 sets

CALISTHENICS

Push-Ups
3 x 25

Abdominal Exercise
(your choice)
3 x 25

SPRINTS

4 X 20 yards
4 X 40 yards
4 X 60 yards

½ mile cool-down run

DAY 3

LEGS

Squats
2 x warm-up
4 x 8

Leg Press (any variety)
1 x warm-up
4 x 8

Leg Extensions
4 x 8

Leg Curls
4 x 8

Calf Raises
(any variety)
1 x warm-up
4 x 8

BICEPS

Barbell Curls
1 x warm-up
4 x 8

Preacher Curls
1 x warm-up
4 x 8

Dumbbell Curls
(any variety)
4 x 8

Forearms
1 x warm-up
3 x 12

Wrist Curls
1 x warm-up
3 x 12

DAY 4

CONDITIONING

2 mile distance run

CALISTHENICS

Squats
2 X 20

Walking Lunges
2 X 20 yards

Calf Raises
2 X 25

SPRINTS

3 x 100 yards
3 X 200 yards

½ mile cool-down run

DAY 5

BACK

Dead Lift
2 x warm-up
4 x 8

Power Clean
1 x warm-up
4 x 8

Bent-over Row
1 x warm-up
4 x 8

Lat Pull-downs
4 x 8

Hyper-extensions
4 x 8

SHOULDERS

Push-press
1 x warm-up
4 x 8

Military Press (or
Behind-the-neck Press)
4 x 8

Lateral Raises
4 x 8

Shrugs
1 x warm-up
4 x 8

Upright Rows
4 x 8

DAY 6

CONDITIONING

½ mile warm-up run

AGILITY DRILLS

Shuttles
3 x 40 yards

Carrioga
3 x 40 yards

Ropes/Tires
3 sets

CALISTHENICS

Push-Ups
3 x 25

Abdominal Exercise
(your choice)
3 x 25

SPRINTS

4 X 20 yards
4 X 40 yards
4 X 60 yards

½ mile cool-down run

WEEK 9

DAY 1

CHEST

Bench Press
1 x Warm Up
12, 10, 8, 6, 4

Incline Bench Press
1 x warm-up
12, 10, 8, 6, 4

Flys (any variation
including machine)
4 x 8

Dumbbell Bench Press
4 x 8

TRICEPS

Triceps Press-downs
(any grip)
1 x warm-up
4 x 8

Triceps Extensions
1 x warm-up
4 x 8

Close Grip Bench
1 x Warm Up
12, 10, 8, 6, 4

DAY 2

CONDITIONING

½ mile warm-up run

AGILITY DRILLS

Shuttles
4 x 40 yards

Carrioga
4 x 40 yards

Ropes/Tires
4 sets

CALISTHENICS

Push-Ups
4 x 25

Abdominal Exercise
(your choice)
4 x 25

SPRINTS

5 X 20 yards
5 X 40 yards
5 X 60 yards

½ mile cool-down run

DAY 3

LEGS

Squats
2 x warm-up
12, 10, 8, 6, 4

Leg Press (any variety)
1 x warm-up
12, 10, 8, 6, 4

Leg Extensions
4 x 8

Leg Curls
4 x 8

Calf Raises
(any variety)
1 x warm-up
4 x 8

BICEPS

Barbell Curls
1 x warm-up
4 x 8

Preacher Curls
1 x warm-up
4 x 8

Dumbbell Curls
4 x 8

Forearms
1 x warm-up
4 x 8

Wrist Curls
1 x warm-up
4 x 8

DAY 4

CONDITIONING

2 ½ mile distance run

CALISTHENICS

Squats
2 X 20

Walking Lunges
2 X 20 yards

Calf Raises
2 X 25

SPRINTS

4 x 100 yards
4 X 200 yards

¼ mile cool-down run

DAY 5

BACK

Dead Lift
2 x warm-up
12, 10, 8, 6, 4

Power Clean
1 x warm-up
12, 10, 8, 6, 4

Bent-over Row
1 x warm-up
4 x 8

Lat Pull-downs
12, 10, 8, 6, 4

Hyper-extensions
4 x 8

SHOULDERS

Push-press
1 x warm-up
12, 10, 8, 6, 4

Military Press (or
Behind-the-neck Press)
4 x 8

Lateral Raises
4 x 8

Shrugs
1 x warm-up
12, 10, 8, 6, 4

Upright Rows
4 x 8

DAY 6

CONDITIONING

½ mile warm-up run

AGILITY DRILLS

Shuttles
4 x 40 yards

Carrioga
4 x 40 yards

Ropes/Tires
4 sets

CALISTHENICS

Push-Ups
4 x 25

Abdominal Exercise
(your choice)
4 x 25

SPRINTS

5 X 20 yards
5 X 40 yards
5 X 60 yards

½ mile cool-down run

WEEK 10

DAY 1	DAY 2	DAY 3

DAY 1

CHEST

Bench Press
1 x Warm Up
12, 10, 8, 6, 4

Incline Bench Press
1 x warm-up
12, 10, 8, 6, 4

Flys (any variation
including machine)
4 x 8

Dumbbell Bench Press
4 x 8

TRICEPS

Triceps Press-downs
(any grip)
1 x warm-up
4 x 8

Triceps Extensions
1 x warm-up
4 x 8

Close Grip Bench
1 x Warm Up
12, 10, 8, 6, 4

DAY 2

CONDITIONING

½ mile warm-up run

AGILITY DRILLS

Shuttles
4 x 40 yards

Carrioga
4 x 40 yards

Ropes/Tires
4 sets

CALISTHENICS

Push-Ups
4 x 25

Abdominal Exercise
(your choice)
4 x 25

SPRINTS

5 X 20 yards
5 X 40 yards
5 X 60 yards

½ mile cool-down run

DAY 3

LEGS

Squats
2 x warm-up
12, 10, 8, 6, 4

Leg Press (any variety)
1 x warm-up
12, 10, 8, 6, 4

Leg Extensions
4 x 8

Leg Curls
4 x 8

Calf Raises
(any variety)
1 x warm-up
4 x 8

BICEPS

Barbell Curls
1 x warm-up
4 x 8

Preacher Curls
1 x warm-up
4 x 8

Dumbbell Curls
4 x 8

Forearms
1 x warm-up
4 x 8

Wrist Curls
1 x warm-up
4 x 8

DAY 4

CONDITIONING

2 ½ mile distance run

CALISTHENICS

Squats
2 X 20

Walking Lunges
2 X 20 yards

Calf Raises
2 X 25

SPRINTS

4 x 100 yards
4 X 200 yards

¼ mile cool-down run

DAY 5

BACK

Dead Lift
2 x warm-up
12, 10, 8, 6, 4

Power Clean
1 x warm-up
12, 10, 8, 6, 4

Bent-over Row
1 x warm-up
4 x 8

Lat Pull-downs
12, 10, 8, 6, 4

Hyper-extensions
4 x 8

SHOULDERS

Push-press
1 x warm-up
12, 10, 8, 6, 4

Military Press (or
Behind-the-neck Press)
4 x 8

Lateral Raises
4 x 8

Shrugs
1 x warm-up
12, 10, 8, 6, 4

Upright Rows
4 x 8

DAY 6

CONDITIONING

½ mile warm-up run

AGILITY DRILLS

Shuttles
4 x 40 yards

Carrioga
4 x 40 yards

Ropes/Tires
4 sets

CALISTHENICS

Push-Ups
4 x 25

Abdominal Exercise
(your choice)
4 x 25

SPRINTS

5 X 20 yards
5 X 40 yards
5 X 60 yards

½ mile cool-down run

WEEK 11

DAY 1

CHEST

Bench Press
1 x Warm Up
12, 10, 8, 6, 4

Incline Bench Press
1 x warm-up
12, 10, 8, 6, 4

Flys (any variation
including machine)
4 x 8

Dumbbell Bench Press
4 x 8

TRICEPS

Triceps Press-downs
(any grip)
1 x warm-up
4 x 8

Triceps Extensions
1 x warm-up
4 x 8

Close Grip Bench
1 x Warm Up
12, 10, 8, 6, 4

DAY 2

CONDITIONING

½ mile warm-up run

AGILITY DRILLS

Shuttles
4 x 40 yards

Carrioga
4 x 40 yards

Ropes/Tires
4 sets

CALISTHENICS

Push-Ups
4 x 25

Abdominal Exercise
(your choice)
4 x 25

SPRINTS

5 X 20 yards
5 X 40 yards
5 X 60 yards

½ mile cool-down run

DAY 3

LEGS

Squats
2 x warm-up
12, 10, 8, 6, 4

Leg Press (any variety)
1 x warm-up
12, 10, 8, 6, 4

Leg Extensions
4 x 8

Leg Curls
4 x 8

Calf Raises
(any variety)
1 x warm-up
4 x 8

BICEPS

Barbell Curls
1 x warm-up
4 x 8

Preacher Curls
1 x warm-up
4 x 8

Dumbbell Curls
4 x 8

Forearms
1 x warm-up
4 x 8

Wrist Curls
1 x warm-up
4 x 8

DAY 4

CONDITIONING

2 ½ mile distance run

CALISTHENICS

Squats
2 X 20

Walking Lunges
2 X 20 yards

Calf Raises
2 X 25

SPRINTS

4 x 100 yards
4 X 200 yards

¼ mile cool-down run

DAY 5

BACK

Dead Lift
2 x warm-up
12, 10, 8, 6, 4

Power Clean
1 x warm-up
12, 10, 8, 6, 4

Bent-over Row
1 x warm-up
4 x 8

Lat Pull-downs
12, 10, 8, 6, 4

Hyper-extensions
4 x 8

SHOULDERS

Push-press
1 x warm-up
12, 10, 8, 6, 4

Military Press (or
Behind-the-neck Press)
4 x 8

Lateral Raises
4 x 8

Shrugs
1 x warm-up
12, 10, 8, 6, 4

Upright Rows
4 x 8

DAY 6

CONDITIONING

½ mile warm-up run

AGILITY DRILLS

Shuttles
4 x 40 yards

Carrioga
4 x 40 yards

Ropes/Tires
4 sets

CALISTHENICS

Push-Ups
4 x 25

Abdominal Exercise
(your choice)
4 x 25

SPRINTS

5 X 20 yards
5 X 40 yards
5 X 60 yards

½ mile cool-down run

WEEK 12

DAY 1	DAY 2	DAY 3

CHEST

Bench Press
1 x Warm Up
12, 10, 8, 6, 4

Incline Bench Press
1 x warm-up
12, 10, 8, 6, 4

Flys (any variation
including machine)
4 x 8

Dumbbell Bench Press
4 x 8

TRICEPS

Triceps Press-downs
(any grip)
1 x warm-up
4 x 8

Triceps Extensions
1 x warm-up
4 x 8

Close Grip Bench
1 x Warm Up
12, 10, 8, 6, 4

CONDITIONING

½ mile warm-up run

AGILITY DRILLS

Shuttles
4 x 40 yards

Carrioga
4 x 40 yards

Ropes/Tires
4 sets

CALISTHENICS

Push-Ups
4 x 25

Abdominal Exercise
(your choice)
4 x 25

SPRINTS

5 X 20 yards
5 X 40 yards
5 X 60 yards

½ mile cool-down run

LEGS

Squats
2 x warm-up
12,10, 8, 6, 4

Leg Press (any variety)
1 x warm-up
12,10, 8, 6, 4

Leg Extensions
4 x 8

Leg Curls
4 x 8

Calf Raises
(any variety)
1 x warm-up
4 x 8

BICEPS

Barbell Curls
1 x warm-up
4 x 8

Preacher Curls
1 x warm-up
4 x 8

Dumbbell Curls
4 x 8

Forearms
1 x warm-up
4 x 8

Wrist Curls
1 x warm-up
4 x 8

DAY 4

CONDITIONING

2 ½ mile distance run

CALISTHENICS

Squats
2 X 20

Walking Lunges
2 X 20 yards

Calf Raises
2 X 25

SPRINTS

4 x 100 yards
4 X 200 yards

¼ mile cool-down run

DAY 5

BACK

Dead Lift
2 x warm-up
12, 10, 8, 6, 4

Power Clean
1 x warm-up
12, 10, 8, 6, 4

Bent-over Row
1 x warm-up
4 x 8

Lat Pull-downs
12, 10, 8, 6, 4

Hyper-extensions
4 x 8

SHOULDERS

Push-press
1 x warm-up
12, 10, 8, 6, 4

Military Press (or
Behind-the-neck Press)
4 x 8

Lateral Raises
4 x 8

Shrugs
1 x warm-up
12, 10, 8, 6, 4

Upright Rows
4 x 8

DAY 6

CONDITIONING

½ mile warm-up run

AGILITY DRILLS

Shuttles
4 x 40 yards

Carrioga
4 x 40 yards

Ropes/Tires
4 sets

CALISTHENICS

Push-Ups
4 x 25

Abdominal Exercise
(your choice)
4 x 25

SPRINTS

5 X 20 yards
5 X 40 yards
5 X 60 yards

½ mile cool-down run

ABOUT THE AUTHORS

Stew Smith is a former Navy SEAL and high school football player. He graduated from the United States Naval Academy in 1991. After graduation, he received orders to SEAL (BUD/S) training.

Stew hails from Live Oak, Florida, home of the Suwannee High School Bulldogs. During his high school athletic career, Stew played football and baseball, ran track, powerlifted and wrestled.

As a member of the Ironman Football Club—where you never leave the field during the entire game—Stew played linebacker, fullback, and on every special team.

Stew's life has been devoted to athletics and exercise. From grade school to SEAL training, he has learned and developed several different regimens. He is the author of several acclaimed workout books including *The Complete Guide to Navy SEAL Fitness* and *Maximum Fitness*.

Stew decided to work with Chris Johnson, a former football player for the University of Pennsylvania, to bring to you this book. This book combines the best of Stew's experiences in the Navy SEALs and on the high school football field with Chris's extensive experience in high school and college football.

Chris Johnson was an All-State Defensive Linemen at North Bergen High School in New Jersey. He was a three-year starter at defensive line for the University of Pennsylvania. Chris was named to the all-Ivy League team twice. He is also a two-time winner of the Chuck Bednarik award for Outstanding Lineman. While Chris played at the University of Pennsylvania the team was undefeated two years running, captured two Ivy League championships, and set a NCAA 1-AA record for consecutive victories.

THE COMPLETE GUIDE TO NAVY SEAL FITNESS

Stewart Smith

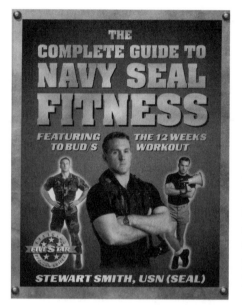

Whether you want to be a Navy SEAL or just look like one...here's your chance! Navy SEALs are ordinary people who do extraordinary jobs. It takes an optimal level of fitness to swim 6 miles, run 15 miles and perform over 150 pull-ups, 400 pushups and 400 sit-ups in one day—but more importantly, it takes motivation and determination to stick with it to the end. If you follow and finish this workout, you will find yourself in the best physical shape of your life!

This new, revised edition brings you: expanded information on what it takes to be a Navy SEAL, including recruitment and preparation; insider's tips to negotiating the famous Navy SEAL obstacle course; new and improved chapters on swimming, running, and nutrition.

The Complete Guide to Navy Seal Fitness is an advanced-level exercise program that teaches running, swimming, rope climbing, stretching, and exercise techniques all in one book. With this program, you will be ready for any military training or physical challenge in the world. Train with the world's fittest and strongest individuals: the US Navy SEALs!

Fully illustrated...packed with photos...just $15.95!

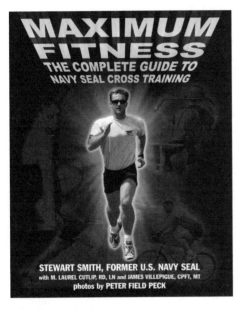

THE BOOK OF SURVIVAL:
THE ORIGINAL GUIDE TO STAYING ALIVE

Anthony Greenbank

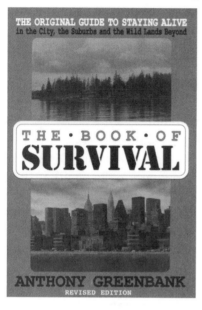

Too lonely...too crowded...too dry...too wet...too bright... too dark... too cold... too hot... too low... too high... too fast... too slow... too full... too empty...

It's never too late, says renowned survival expert Anthony Greenbank, if "whoever faces catastrophe takes a deep breath and makes up his mind to have a really determined go at beating the odds."

If you're caught in a calamity, the advice given in **The Book of Survival** can save your life. The suggestions are organized so you will remember them in a flash of cold clarity at the right moment. Forewarned is forearmed, and this book equips you with the knowledge necessary to fend off a stick-up artist, work out of ropes that bind you, use your facial muscles to prevent frostbite, start a fire with your camera, vault over an oncoming car, improvise a stove and a tent and much, much more.

The Book of Survival is a textbook for non-heroes, presenting a practical program for survival under any circumstances. It a manual to read, re-read, remember—and give to your loved ones.

300 pages...illustrated...essential...just $14.95!

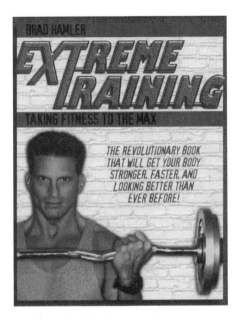

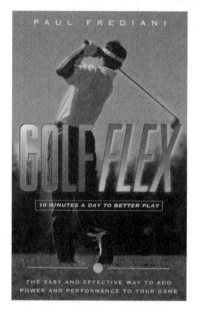